WHAT OTHERS ARE SAYING ABOUT "TAKE BACK YOUR BIRTH"

"Lynn delivers a powerful critique of the standard American model of birth and raises the bar on how we define success in childbirth. She inspires her readers to reevaluate their priorities for their own childbearing experiences and provides practical tips for preparing to achieve one's ideal birth. Lynn's words shine with her passion for mothers, babies, and families. She is a beacon, illuminating the way for couples who seek a better way to birth." -Lilah Monger, mother of eleven, Instructor at Ancient Art Midwifery Institute

"It is very comforting to know that the seed we have kept warm in our hands, in the depths of our souls, is finally emerging and with Lynn's 'Take Back Your Birth: Inspiration for Expectant Moms,' you can now join the migration of women with wings and birth without reservations, with your book displacing 'birth fear' with truth and trust in her own body, because she desires what she knows is best for her baby." -Lynn Reed, Trust Birth facilitator and Founder of Better Augusta Birth Experience (BABE)

"Ms. Griesemer offers a refreshing perspective on childbirth, marriage, and family life. A wonderful book for exploring a variety of loving options and thinking 'outside the box' for the best possible birth for you and your family. -Fiona Grant-Endsley, mother of three happy homeborn children

TAKE BACK YOUR BIRTH

INSPIRATION FOR EXPECTANT MOMS

Lynn M. Griesemer

Terra Publishing, Tampa, FL
ISBN: 0-9661066-4-4 and ISBN 13: 978-0-9661066-4-0

Library of Congress Control Number: 2018900324

Cover design: Melanie Griesemer. www.melaniegriesemer.com
Photo: provided by Devon Roe. www.DevonRoePhotography.com

In some cases, the pronoun "he" is used as a generic pronoun.

Do you want free books? Lynn M. Griesemer is giving away free books as part of her "Your Marriage Matters" series. These titles are exclusive for members of her free Your Marriage Matters (YMM) Movement Group. Visit www.marriagecoachlynn.com to receive your first book in the series, "Make Your Marriage Great: Clean of Heart."

DISCLAIMER

This book is designed to provide information about the subject matter covered. It is sold with the understanding that the publisher and author are not engaged in rendering any psychological and medical advice or services. If expert assistance is desired or required, the services of a competent professional should be sought.

The purpose of this book is to share and encourage. The publisher and author shall have neither liability nor responsibility to any person or entity with respect to any loss or damage caused or alleged to be caused directly or indirectly by the information contained in this book.

DEDICATION

to women in their childbearing years: choose wisely

CALL TO ACTION

We are at a crossroads regarding the manner in which babies are born. On the one hand, medicated and surgical deliveries remain high, yet at the same time, there is a growing number of homebirths.

Far too many women take for granted the American way of labor and delivery, and end up having a birth experience that leaves them disappointed. Our culture focuses on the senses, materialism, and the physical – what we can measure and see. What is neglected are the emotional, mental, and unseen dimensions of childbirth. We will not experience childbirth to its fullest capacity if we forget about these aspects.

Let us draw our attention to what REALLY matters, and that is, the feminine experience of childbirth that leaves you fulfilled. "Take Back Your Birth" is an invitation to expectant mothers to examine their philosophy of birth. In it you'll find criticism of the excessive use of technology and machines, but nestled among the pages of this book, you will find encouragement and practical tips for an autonomous birth.

ADDITIONAL ENCOURAGEMENT can be found by visiting www.unassistedhomebirth.com and www.marriagecoachlynn.com

CONTENTS

CONTENTS

MY STORY

I am the mother of six children. My first four children were born in the hospital between 1988 and 1993 and by the time we were ready to welcome our youngest two children, we chose to have them at home, with no doctor or midwife. I was fed up with the American way of delivering babies. I was in excellent health and most of my babies were born within three hours of the onset of labor. I had minimal medical intervention for the first four children, but my intuition told me that something wasn't quite right.

A lot wasn't quite right. I was coached in pushing out my first baby, told to lay still while the doctor "did a little cut" (episiotomy) and directed me in giving birth. He told me he almost hit a deer on the way to the hospital as he sped to get there after midnight, half asleep. He practically blamed me for interrupting his sleep. Our baby was delivered and whisked away for an hour for measurements. The doctor, in a hurry to finish, mashed aggressively on my abdomen to get the placenta out minutes after our son was born.

The birth of our second baby was like an assembly line delivery, with five or six women left alone to labor in their individual rooms. The doctor went from patient to patient, like a juggler keeping tennis balls in the air. At one point, the doctor seemed bored and told my husband to go downstairs and get a sandwich in the cafeteria to pass the time. The hallway was filled with the sounds of heartbeats thumping from the electronic fetal monitors. The nurse was coaching me how to give birth and strangers came and went in and out of my room.

I noticed a man in scrubs with a black bag and asked, "Who's that and what is he doing here?" I knew beyond a shadow of a doubt that I would not want or need any medication, but by law, they told me, an anesthesiologist had to be on call in the room, "just in case." The bill for that one-minute intrusive witnessing of my private birth event? $100.00. It was 1990.

Things happened during my births whether or not I wanted them to happen.

Our third baby made her entrance into the world within ten minutes of arrival at the hospital and there was very little time for anyone to patronize me or persuade me to have medical interventions. However, the attitude exhibited by the doctor and some staff members afterwards was businesslike. It felt sterile and insincere. It was difficult being in an environment while one of the most intense, meaningful events of my life was taking place.

Back to the hospital again for our fourth baby's birth. I didn't know any better. I had no social network of women friends who did anything different than select the most popular doctor in town and the nearest hospital. Because I was in the hospital for four hours before our daughter was born, they had time to mess with me. My amniotic sac was broken, internal and external fetal monitors were installed, and Pitocin was given to me to "speed up the labor." I seemed to have no choice. I was a slab of meat and this was the protocol.

Christina was born with a scab on her upper forehead, near the hairline and I asked both the Ob/Gyn and the pediatrician if the internal fetal monitor could have caused the scab. "Oh no," they said, "It's a congenital birth mark." I believed them at the time.

I told my husband a few years later that if we had another child, I would like to look into a homebirth. Intuitively, I knew I would enjoy a homebirth. When I got pregnant with our fifth child, I found the right resources and we chose to have the baby at home.

Again, in 2002, we chose to stay home to give birth. The birth experiences of our two youngest children were empowering and inspiring, natural and "real." Everything flowed and seemed right.

In 1996, I began encouraging other couples to consider unassisted birth and in 1998, I published "Unassisted Homebirth: An Act of Love." Since then, many changes have taken place in the birth world, and not all have been positive. It is true that many more women are choosing to give birth at home, but at the same time, medical childbirth is on the rise.

This book is for women in the childbearing years who want something much, much better than hospitals can offer. I wish I had a book like this when I was pregnant with my first child. I would have taken a completely different path for the births of my first four children. Please consider your options and choose wisely. I am dedicated to helping couples build strong marriages and pursue more autonomy in their birth experiences.

Visit my websites for support:

www.unassistedhomebirth.com
www.marriagecoachlynn.com.

INTRODUCTION

You can have the birth of your dreams if you believe you can and if you strive for it. It takes courage, education, confidence and mental and physical determination to have a birth you will cherish for the rest of your life. If the outcome does not result in your "dream," at least you will have done everything possible to make it the best it can be.

The purpose of this book is to encourage you to make choices that are best for you. I will not rehash all of the factual details related to childbirth; there is a plethora of facts and statistics available for you to access, and technological changes are ongoing. Instead, I will mention some basics as I present my opinions and reasoning, with the main objective of inspiring and encouraging you to make your birth experience far more satisfying than it currently is for many couples.

A major theme of this book is feminine empowerment, with a strong bias toward natural homebirth. In my situation, I gravitated toward unassisted homebirth, or birth without a midwife, attendant, or doctor. This book is for any woman who desires a dignified and satisfying childbirth experience, regardless of location or medication choices. If you are truly educated and make decisions that you are comfortable with, then your birth can be the beautiful experience it was meant to be. It is mainly about your inner preparation, something which has been sorely lacking in our culture for decades.

You may notice some repetition or overlap among chapters. That is intentional since each chapter can stand alone. You may also notice a negative tone at times. It is important to shine the light on problems within the system in order to see that change is needed. In doing so, the negative facets must be discussed and analyzed.

Women do not realize that they will revisit their birth experience for the rest of their lives. Memories are triggered by certain events or a mother may be reminded of her birth experience each time her child celebrates a birthday.

It is the philosophy of birth that needs to undergo examination. Once we arrive at our philosophy of birth, we can plan for action. However, be aware of following through on YOUR preferences as opposed to being influenced by other women's narratives. Their birth story is not your birth story.

Philosophies and beliefs about birth can change. Successful childbirth is not about some self-centered approach to birth or searching for an orgasmic birth, but it is striving for what is best for the mother, baby and family unit. It is about purposely seeking the safest and most satisfying situation possible. It is about looking toward an event fully prepared, expecting the best.

Birth is much more than a medical event. It is possibly THE highlight of a woman's sexuality. When you are able to tap into your emotional, spiritual, mental and physical power, childbirth can become an opportunity for true, long-lasting joy.

"Realize that you cannot hurry success any more than the lilies of the field can bloom before their season."   -Og Mandino

PART I: BIRTH IN AMERICA: WHAT'S WRONG?

CHAPTER 1: WHY WE DON'T NEED EXPERTS

When it comes to birth, we don't need experts. Childbirth is not a complicated process and the majority of the population could birth without so-called experts. Unfortunately, many women refuse to believe that they are physically capable of birthing outside a hospital, without a doctor or midwife. Because they cling to firmly held birth beliefs, there is little hope for changing the hearts and minds of women who depend upon experts to assist or bring about the birth of their baby.

WHO ARE THE EXPERTS?

We could say that experts are those who have received formal training and experience (such as a doctor, midwife, medical professional) as well as anyone who positions themselves to make someone think they hold the answers and solutions to a particular problem or situation. An expert and someone who seeks the services of that expert are not in an equal position. Therefore, the person seeking the opinion or treatment is in a submissive or subservient role to the expert.

WHAT DO THE EXPERTS DO FOR US?

Experts in a chosen field have the ability to help those truly in need. We should be grateful for the contribution experts have made as far as research, expertise for those who need it, and information that can be used by the masses. Alternative childbirth researchers estimate that approximately 5% of the population truly need C-sections. Others with medical problems might require an expert during the prenatal or postpartum period and many argue that perception plays a large part in the REAL need for medical advice or treatment.

What are the experts motivated by? Motives may include: money, research, ego, pushing science to its extreme, the assumption that patients are in misery and need relief via drugs, successful business practices and reputation. Experts' priorities are most likely not the same as your priorities. Pleasing the hospital or insurance company, striving for a higher paycheck, and avoiding litigation are not putting the customers' needs first. A doctor who is first and foremost thinking of litigation means that patients are potential enemies.

Will the experts share secrets for success? Can you really count on the experts? How many times have you known women to arrive for their birth and find that another doctor (not of their choice) announces that he or she will be their birth attendant? How many women do you know end up getting added "extras" (such as an epidural, Pitocin, internal monitor or a C-section) during the final moments of birth, especially when they've communicated other intentions to the experts they hired?

Experts may not want you becoming a mini-expert to make their job easier. As they see it, they've got a job to do and are well qualified to do it. Midwives and other birth professionals bring their fears and past experience to your birth. We are the sum total of our experiences and we cannot be sure whether or not the expertise coming our way is the kind of competence we will need for our unique birth.

WHY DO WE SEEK EXPERTS?

EXPERTS AS PROVIDERS. We seek experts because we believe that they can give us something we don't have, be it information, treatment or equipment. Many American women perceive childbirth to be complex, requiring certain equipment or resources.

COMPETENCE. We seek experts when we think something is too complex or specialized; we are searching for a highly skilled or trained professional.

AVOIDANCE OF PAIN IS STRONGER THAN THE DESIRE FOR PLEASURE. Many women perceive that childbirth will always be excruciatingly painful and that we want to avoid it at all costs, especially by using drugs during labor and delivery.

SOCIALIZATION / CUSTOM. "We might as well go to an obstetrician because that's what the rest of the culture does." Social conditioning fails us because we're taught to look up to the experts, while disregarding our thoughts, desires and intuition. "Show respect. Do not offend. Be conformant."

My sister once asked me a very insightful question: "Doctors have had many years of experience to build on. Don't you think they have ironed out a lot of learning to bring themselves to a point of almost pure expertise when it comes to childbirth?" The implied message was: "How could I disregard the already existing perfect knowledge and choose to serve as my own expert?" I am also reminded of the midwife who once said, "There's more to birth than just reading a few books and having a positive attitude. Women need a caring, loving, skilled attendant at their births."

I have come to this conclusion: Let's assume that every goal of a birth outcome is for a healthy baby. Picture train tracks. Train tracks have two parallel rails, separated and linked together by railroad ties, which run perpendicular to those tracks. The medical profession represents one side of the train tracks and alternative birthers, the other. We are all seeking the same destination, but we are getting there in our own separate ways. Occasionally we share information. Unfortunately, alternative birthers are not given as much credibility as the "professionals." Who's to say that one person or method is more valid than another?

WHAT HAPPENS TO THOSE WHO EMPLOY EXPERTS?

For starters, the mother, father and baby are not in control of their own birth. The doctor is the problem-solver and ultimately, the patient must obey instructions. Patients may get bullied into taking drugs, tests, even having an abortion. If pregnancy is not desired, artificial birth control is expected of any woman who consults a typical gynecologist. A few doctors have proclaimed to me that the pill is "God's gift to women" and often do not know or care about natural fertility methods.

Well-baby visits make you think you need an expert to give his seal of approval for your child's development. When we question convention or the experts, we are sometimes treated as if we are unwise or wrong. Parents who decide to forego vaccinations for their children are often seen as a health threat, uneducated or rebellious. In extreme cases, the Department of Social Services poses as experts by intervening in cases where it thinks parents are neglectful or non-conformant.

If we go to the hospital for birth, knowing that we are relinquishing our power and deliberately choosing to ignore our intuition and knowledge, we are failing ourselves by not being true to ourselves. What we are doing is not giving ourselves much credit and passing ourselves to someone else to take care of us. We set up an unequal relationship and we tip the balance scale in favor of the experts who will make all final decisions. Those who turn to experts throughout pregnancy and birth must now find new experts for childrearing as well as other aspects of their lives.

Women need to take back their power. The most troubling fact of all is that women are not taught or encouraged to go deep inside themselves and birth with strength and confidence. We need a strong mental attitude to give birth; every cell in our bodies and every ounce of energy is required to birth a new being into existence. And what do the experts want to do? – lay us down, examine us, drug us, hook us up to electrical equipment, and tell us to perform within a certain time-frame. We are tampered with when we go to experts.

WHAT WE CAN DO

It is crucial to wean ourselves from experts by gaining confidence and knowledge, which diminishes fear and helplessness. We can adapt whatever parts of medical research that can help us achieve a successful birth. Although I do not desire a midwife during birth, I found many good ideas from Sheila Kitzinger's books, especially about what to do in emergencies or tough situations. Today's Millennial has so much information at her fingertips. Videos and on-line communities are just one easy click away.

There will always be periods of doubt while preparing for the birth of a baby in a hospital setting, as well as an unassisted homebirth. Many of us doubt and question many aspects of our lives; it's a natural part of living. Even though we may become knowledgeable about childbirth, we must be open to new beliefs and perceptions. Some women take good quality birth classes or talk with those who have had satisfying, unmedicated births, yet they opt for an epidural or end up with a C-section. It's partly because they have not successfully worked through fears, inhibitions, and long held beliefs. They will not release the chains that bind them because it's easier to cling to comfortable assumptions than it is to venture into the unknown. All the education in the world will not change firmly held beliefs.

We need to build confidence to move forward in life so that we do not depend on experts, because for most births, we're better off without the experts. Mistakes, harm and even deaths occur during the millions of hospital births each year. Experts are helpful, but they can also fail and disappoint us every day.

WHAT WE GAIN

By becoming our own expert at birth, we become more intimately involved in life and as a family member. Becoming an expert enables us to be more independent and self-sufficient. This makes us less draining on society; we won't need others for something we can do ourselves. When we see ourselves as experts, we develop competence and additional problem solving abilities; we increase confidence in ourselves and trust in the birth process.

Satisfying moments in life where we did not employ experts inspire a sense of pride. Sometimes our plan doesn't come to fruition and must come to a point of acceptance. When we view an experience as a failure, we struggle with guilt, blame and self-worth issues. All of these things move us towards introspection and a fuller, richer life.

The greatest possible gain from childbirth is intangible. It is often overlooked by medicalized birth, but extremely important to relationships. And that is the opportunity for couples to solidify their union with each other. Most newlyweds enter marriage making a commitment to each other for a lifetime. Rather than form a union with a doctor or midwife that is the equivalent of an impersonal, casual, short-lived affair, couples need to look no farther than themselves for a birth that is almost always safe, joyous and everlasting. How can a husband and wife achieve a bond with each other at birth with obstetricians and nurses directing the event during a medicalized birth? It's possible and a lot of inner work must be done to ensure an intimate birth experience.

"Your future emanates totally and absolutely from your present mental attitude." – Mark Victor Hansen

"If you are distressed by anything external, the pain is not due to the thing itself, but to your estimate of it; and this you have the power to revoke at any moment." –Marcus Aurelius

CHAPTER 2: NINE MYTHS OF CHILDBIRTH

(1) Pregnancy and childbirth are abnormal.
(2) Technology always benefits pregnancy and childbirth.
(3) Birth is usually unsafe: death is a possibility.
(4) Birth is an emergency.
(5) Professionals are needed to deliver babies.
(6) Birth is unbearably painful.
(7) Childbirth is scary.
(8) The C-section was necessary.
(9) Women need episiotomies, especially with their firstborn.

Birth is a simple process, but because of our fears, we do not believe that birth is uncomplicated and safe. Perhaps there were problems that warranted specific attention. What originally started out as genuine concerns have been embellished or exaggerated. Some myths are perpetuated by those who know the truth. Misconceptions that have gained momentum must be challenged by educated and courageous people in order for change to occur.

Myths come from misinformation and ignorance. Actions are based on beliefs that can become habits. When cultures adopt commonly held beliefs and habits, they influence birth practices. The nine myths of childbirth are an example of "cultural conformity," the major stumbling block to change.

MYTH (1) PREGNANCY AND BIRTH ARE ABNORMAL

Many physicians and patients consider pregnancy and birth an abnormality or illness. With their words and images, a significant number of journalists and filmmakers perpetuate the idea that pregnancy and birth are distasteful. We are taught that the goal of pregnancy is to treat any discomfort and rid the body of the abnormal, ill condition.

When the fetus is seen as a foreign intruder, it is hard to rejoice about the pregnancy, making childbirth thought of as painful and unnatural, as if the body were not designed to give birth. Those who believe this myth then become overly cautious and try not to cause further disruption. When the mother is taught that she must accommodate this burdensome state, she then begins to view what should be a time filled with joy and anticipation as a personal sacrifice, a mere condition threatening her lifestyle.

Some women avoid physical activity, sexual pleasure and make other changes because they think pregnancy and birth are abnormal. Sadly, I've known many women who said they hated being pregnant and couldn't wait to return to "normal."

Abnormal cases require professionals to solve problems and develop treatments. They seem to test the limits of science by looking for problems. Since everyone has minor discomforts, such as heartburn, nausea, or swelling, it is easy to label every pregnancy as problematic. Typical doctor appointments during pregnancy focus on abnormalities through various tests and screenings. The abnormalities of pregnancy and birth include not only rare defects, but man-imposed interference such as fertility drugs and vacuum extraction deliveries.

MYTH (2) TECHNOLOGY ALWAYS BENEFITS PREGNANCY AND CHILDBIRTH

People agree that more is better and that we should have as much technology as possible so that we will be equipped for emergencies. But what often happens is that the technology that was once designed for abnormal cases gets used for routine cases; it gets overused or misused.

I have seen a rise in the use of technology since my first pregnancy in 1988. Rather than one ultrasound appointment, some practices recommend three during the pregnancy and it is not uncommon for women to receive between four and six ultrasound scans per pregnancy!

Blood is tested for HIV and sexually transmitted infections, something monogamous couples do not have to worry about. Many practices suggest amniocentesis testing simply because a woman is over 35. The AFP (Alpha-fetoprotein) test is routinely used to determine abnormality. Doctors admit the high rate of "false positives" even though women are told that it is taken so that they can "mentally prepare" for a less than normal child or so that specialists can be on-hand at the birth. By high, I mean that of the 5% of tests that are deemed positive, 90% of women go on to deliver a healthy, normal child. The high rate of inaccuracies creates needless worrying, further testing or an abortion-decision in a society that demands perfection.

Technology is available in the hospital in case there are problems. For the majority of women who do not have problematic births, technology is employed routinely; there are big profits to be made. Medical professionals and the general population assume that technology is almost always beneficial. It is, when it is truly needed. However, the misuse of technology can result in unnecessary inductions and C-sections, occasionally resulting in premature babies.

People imagine birth without technology. They assume childbirth methods were primitive and dangerous. The danger was caused not by the absence of technology, but by inferior personal hygiene and other factors. Perhaps there were more deaths without technology, but far too many infant deaths today are caused by advanced science. Says Dr. David Stewart, cofounder of NAPSAC (International Association of Parents and Professionals for Safe Alternatives in Childbirth): "Since 1940 at least a million babies have died in American hospitals who would have lived were it not for the doctor dominated maternity system that dictates the Standards for American Childbirth."

The United States is one of the lowest ranking modern countries in maternal and neonatal safety in the world, which is surprising for one of the most technologically advanced countries. This tells me that something is lacking with the way technology is administered during pregnancy and birth and is not an indication that American women's bodies are ill equipped to give birth.

During delivery, an internal fetal monitor is commonly used, in addition to the external fetal monitor (EFM). EFMs have not been proven to increase the safety of birth. In addition to restricting the woman's movement during labor, EFMs have been known to have inaccuracies. Dr. Edward H. Hon invented the electronic fetal monitor and intended it to be used only during difficult labors. Now, the EFM is used routinely, requiring the woman to be in a restricted and often uncomfortable position during labor. The EFM is used to make important decisions, which often lead to unnecessary interventions. "Oh, no, the baby is in distress; we must do an emergency C-section."

Here is what Hon stated about his own invention several years after its widespread implementation: "Not all patients should be electronically monitored. Most women in labor may be much better off at home than in the hospital with the electronic fetal monitor."

There are at least three opinions on the safety of ultrasound. Many say it is perfectly safe, while others say that we don't know the effects of ultrasound. Some cite evidence that ultrasound is dangerous. The American College of

Obstetrics and Gynecology, the American College of Radiology, and the U.S. Preventive Services Task Force all recommend AGAINST routine ultrasound screening of low-risk pregnancies.

Technology is beneficial when it is used to aid difficult situations where it is impossible to rely on human means. However, technology is often used to direct the birth event. And remember, overemphasis upon technology results in a move away from human contact and natural aspects of childbirth. Natural childbirth gives women the pleasure of experiencing a key aspect of their sexuality in a fully conscious, alert state of mind and body.

MYTH (3) BIRTH IS USUALLY UNSAFE; DEATH IS A POSSIBILITY

Anything can go wrong with the mother and the baby. Death may occur during childbirth. People obsess about a remote possibility, but their fears do not reflect reality. Generations have managed to reproduce without a massive infant or mother mortality rate.

The belief that birth is unsafe has contributed to current obstetrical practices. To ensure that birth will be safer, doctors feel the need to manage birth in a controlled, predictable manner. The baseline for a successful birth is that the mother and baby emerge from the ordeal alive. Many people believe birth must be attended by a physician in a hospital to prevent against the possibility of death. While people are concentrating on all the things that can go wrong, they cannot see all that is going well.

It is possible that the same group of people who worry about death in childbirth do not fret about the possibility that their plane will crash, that they will contract a disease from store-bought food or that they will get into a fatal car accident. While death is a highly unlikely result of childbirth, it is more common in hospitals than at home. Newborns exhibit breathing difficulties more frequently after medicated hospital births than they do in unmedicated births at home. Hospital nurseries are filled with many more unhealthy babies, percentage wise, than babies born at home.

"Compared to home-born babies, hospital-born babies are six times more likely to suffer distress during labor, eight times more likely to need resuscitation, four times more likely to become infected, 30 times more likely to suffer permanent injury, and their mothers are three times more likely to hemorrhage. The high risk is in the hospital." (Balizet 1996: 141)

Today's Millennial Mom's baby is faced with compromised infant health due to an excessive induction rate. Alternative health practitioners caution against induction before 41 or 42 weeks gestation.

Whether they are born in a hospital or at home, the majority of babies are born alive and healthy.

MYTH (4) BIRTH IS AN EMERGENCY

If birth is an emergency, why do some doctors show up for delivery at the last possible minute? The labor and delivery staff in a hospital calmly go about their business while the mother is waiting around to deliver her baby. It is not until the baby is about to be born that the birthing room dramatics begin. The doctor may order commands when to push. His instruments are wheeled over to him and the anesthesiologist suddenly appears. The entire delivery room staff seems to care and act as if a major crisis is about to occur, making the mother feel as if it is an emergency.

"The crisis nature of birth was retained from the medical model, and childbirth, as practiced by the Lamaze, prepared-childbirth instructors, continued to be defined in terms of medicine rather than motherhood. It is the homebirth movement that presented the genuine challenges to the medical model." (Rothman 1994: 94)

The out-of-hospital births which get media attention are those that are not planned. Everyone has seen or heard of the news headline where a couple were speeding to the hospital and had the baby in their car. Oh how relieved we are to discover that things turned out favorably. People expect a major problem in the absence of a professional and attribute success to luck. Our biology works in certain ways for certain reasons; there is no luck about it.

MYTH (5) PROFESSIONALS ARE NEEDED TO DELIVER BABIES

If birth is abnormal, unsafe and an emergency, then a professional must manage the situation. "Birth moved into hospitals in large part because doctors believed it was a surgical event." (Rothman 1994: 284). The propaganda has continued for decades and we still pay homage to the man in the white coat. Patients allow doctors to make many decisions for them and submit to C-sections and unnecessary interventions.

Obstetricians and midwives ordinarily approach childbirth with a businesslike, matter-of-factness. It is not unusual for birth to become a mechanical-surgical event, complete with medication and physical restraint. Birth decisions are based on the convenience of the doctor rather than the parents. When you sign up with a doctor or midwife, you are signing onto their regulations and restrictions; their choice of hospital comes before yours.

Many people believe that the doctor or midwife has the best interests of the patient in mind. This may or may not be true, depending on the particular attendant. Patients believe that because they pay experts, the experts' judgment is flawless. Many women do not see themselves, but their doctor or midwife as the center of birth. Although many may not agree, professionals are not NEEDED to bring about a birth. Most babies emerge when they are ready.

MYTH (6) BIRTH IS UNBEARABLY PAINFUL

Rather than prepare for birth naturally and lovingly, women fear a big baby passing through the vagina. The assumption that childbirth is extremely painful is accepted as a fact and since it is perceived as true, the experience of pain often accompanies the birth. The father is asked to be distant from the whole experience and to focus on trivial breathing exercises with his wife. Many couples attend weekly lessons on how to breathe, only to forget them when they get to the delivery room.

Related to this myth is the idea that you need drugs to make it through the delivery. Drugs are readily available and can alleviate any amount of pain a woman may have. Sedatives and narcotic drugs are used to squelch complaints.

Physical pain intensifies not only because of the actual pain experienced, but also based on a woman's perception, ability to cope with pain, and level of emotional support. Hospitals do not provide much emotional support. People she has never met before will be present at the birth, making sure she is hooked up to the EFM. On a busy shift, the nurse will have to go from room to room to check the EFM results, leaving the woman alone to stare at the clock.

Birth is defined by pain: what to do about it rather than how to avoid it or how to work in synchronization with it. Without drugs, the first stage of labor may be more painful, but the second stage, the pushing phase, will be less painful and more manageable by the woman. All a mother really needs is reassurance and human compassion.

Fear and pain go together when it comes to childbirth. Grantly Dick-Read said that fear influences the muscles which cause tension and anxiety. Pain intensifies and doctors are there to relieve that pain. "Civilization and culture have brought influences to bear upon the minds of women which have introduced justifiable fears and anxieties concerning labor. The more cultured the races of the earth have become, so much the more dogmatic have they been in pronouncing childbirth to be a painful and dangerous ordeal...If fear can be eliminated, pain will cease." (Dick-Read 1959: 6)

"Of all our physical functions, only lovemaking is as much influenced by thoughts and emotions as labor. The way the mother thinks and feels affects the way she gives birth." (Jones 1987: 5)

MYTH (7) CHILDBIRTH IS SCARY

Through the birth experience we come to terms with who we are and how we deal with stress and uncertainty, because birth is an opportunity to test our physical and emotional limits. While many people live their lives with a sense of busyness, some flee from the self, some avoid spending time alone by engaging in frenetic activity. It is in the quiet moments that spiritual and psychological truths are discovered. The more self-acceptance and self-awareness we have, the greater likelihood for a calm, happy life.

Fear comes from an inability to trust the body and nature, and women's magazine sales thrive on an inferiority complex which leads women to think they need to aspire to some ideal body. The pressure to improve weight and muscle tone is not motivated so much by health reasons as it is by psychological reasons. Indeed, some people do not even enjoy their pregnancies and at the eighth or ninth month, they are looking forward to having the baby so that they can shed those "unsightly pounds and get back to normal."

A poor body image contributes to inhibitions, often accompanied by shyness, modesty, and embarrassment. When a woman expresses fear to her doctor, she is questioning her confidence and ability. Many doctors are unlikely to ask a woman why she doubts herself or reassure her that there is no reason to fear birth. Instead, doctors often accept the woman's self-assessment as fact. They do not help build a positive body image for pregnancy and birth, but rather let the fear spread into pain and treat the pain in the delivery room.

Insecurity contributes to the myth that childbirth is scary, so drugs are used to minimize fear and inhibitions as well to reduce perceived or actual pain. Not only do women miss out on satisfying birth experiences, but low self-confidence carries over to the beginning days and months of parenting, leading to insecurities about parenting.

If we think and act as if birth is scary, we will ignore our inner intelligence, which tells us that birth is not to be feared. We will rely upon experts, never realizing that we are experts.

MYTH (8) THE C-SECTION WAS NECESSARY

"Thank God for the C-section. I needed it." Maybe so and maybe not. Although some women are grateful for the special medical attention that brought about the birth of their baby, others are disappointed with themselves or their doctors. If you are uneasy about a previous C-section, check out the International Cesarean Awareness Network (ICAN) for information, support, and a directory of local chapters.

Many people accept the idea that every birth is a potential (or probable) C-section. A baby in "distress," in breech position, or too big to come out vaginally often prompt C-sections. New moms are grateful for the C-section of their nine pound baby because they are fearful when they imagine a vaginal birth of a big baby. Others are relieved to have a C-section when the EFM reveals that the baby's heart rate stopped or that labor was not progressing.

Research indicates that the true need for C-sections applies to five percent of the pregnant population, but (depending on the doctor and hospital), one-third of women end up with C-sections. My friend told me about an American hospital with a 50% C-section rate. Some hospitals in Brazil have an 85% C-section rate.

I want to encourage you to do everything in your power to avoid a C-section and to be certain that you are in the 5% of women who physiologically need a C-section. I do not have time here to elaborate, but the research you will discover will clearly reveal that a vaginal birth is superior to a C-section. And, it is a sad commentary on our culture that there is still rampant fear and avoidance by many OB/Gyn practices to dissuade women from having a VBAC for subsequent births. I know hundreds of women who were misled into preparing for a VBAC, and during the last week of pregnancy or in the delivery room, they were provided an excuse to consent to another C-section.

"The medical establishment states to the public, as well as to the students in their medical schools, that the increased cesarean rates are for the benefit of mothers, babies and families. The data do not support this claim." (Stewart: 1997: 56). Many C-sections are preventable. Proper prenatal habits, combined with assertiveness on the part of the birthing couple, an unhurried attendant, and avoidance of elective medication may help you avoid a C-section.

If you've come to the conclusion that your C-section was unnecessary, I urge you to face the issue, rather than bury any pain you may have about that birth. Healing and acceptance can be difficult, but ignoring and avoiding usually result in long term effects.

MYTH (9) WOMEN NEED EPISIOTOMIES, ESPECIALLY WITH THE FIRSTBORN

Thankfully, the episiotomy rate has diminished to 10% over the past few decades. I commend the medical establishment for progressing in the right direction. While some episiotomies are needed, others are performed because of the preference or routine of the doctor. The "need" for an episiotomy is, after all, determined by the doctor. Many women tear even after they have had an episiotomy and many others have long and difficult recoveries from episiotomies, possibly worse recoveries than if they had torn.

Women are not taught perineal massage and do not have warm water with oil applied to the perineum to prevent tearing. Lying in a supported supine position in the birthing room does not help matters. In fact, many childbirth educators have presented data which show that a squatting position at delivery reduces tearing by an additional ten percent. If women knew how to prepare their bodies (during the prenatal period) and followed a few simple procedures during birth, they would not need an episiotomy. See Chapter 3 for tips.

HOW YOU CAN HAVE A SATISFYING BIRTH IN SPITE OF THE MYTHS:

(1) Change what you think about birth and you will change your experience of it.

(2) Ignore pessimists and complainers. Surround yourself with people who have had fulfilling births.

(3) Do not allow anyone to define what childbirth should entail. You can choose how you want your birth to go by setting goals, planning, and asserting your desires in the delivery room.

(4) Arrive at the hospital well into labor. You may feel more comfort (and less pain) at home. There will be less time for overuse of technology.

(5) Realize that the birthing room drama is often exaggerated and that most births are not true emergencies.

"Error will prevail when truth is obscured by darkness. Seek the truth and banish error from the mind." – Lynn M. Griesemer

"Things are never as good as they seem or as bad as they seem. The business of life is nothing but a business of momentum. Stay inspired – don't get complacent during good times and don't doubt yourself during bad times." – Art Williams

References:

Arms, Suzanne. "Immaculate Deception: A New Look at Women and Childbirth in America." 1975. Houghton Mifflin, Co., Boston, MA.

Armstrong, Penny, C.N.M. and Feldman, Sheryl. "A Wise Birth: Bringing Together the Best of Natural Childbirth with Modern Medicine." 1990, William Morrow & Co., Inc., NY.

Balizet, Carol. "Born in Zion: A Journal of True Adventures in Learning the Faithfulness of God." 1992. Christ Center Publishing International, Euless, TX.

Dick-Read, Grantly, M.D. "Childbirth Without Fear: The Principles and Practice of Natural Childbirth." (2nd ed.) 1959. Harper & Row Publishers, NY.

Griesemer, Lynn M. "Unassisted Homebirth: An Act of Love." 1998. Terra Publishing, Tampa, FL.

Jones, Carl. "Mind Over Labor: A Breakthrough Guide to Giving Birth." 1988. Viking Penguin, Inc., NY, NY.

Rothman, Barbara Katz. "In Labor: Women and Power in the Birthplace." 1982. W.W. Norton& Co., NY, NY.

Stewart, David, Ph.D. "The Five Standards for Safe Childbearing." 1997. NAPSAC International, Marble Hill, MO.

CHAPTER 3: TEN SECRETS YOUR OBSTETRICIAN WON'T TELL YOU

(1) How to avoid an episiotomy.
(2) How to avoid a C-section.
(3) Major decisions are based on inconclusive tests and technology.
(4) Risks and effects of legal drugs during labor.
(5) His goals and your goals are different.
(6) Birth is a straightforward, uncomplicated process.
(7) He may not have expertise in normal, natural birth.
(8) You are not in full control of your own birth.
(9) Mental imagery is extremely important for birth.
(10) How to have a successful birth.

Childbirth is a multi-billion dollar industry in which paid experts are trained to detect and react to problems. Birth is designed to occur naturally, but often results in a delivery which is far from natural. Obstetricians may not tell their patients the ten secrets for several reasons – and these are generalities. (1) doctors act in ways that will justify the need for their expertise, (2) doctors want to put their medical training to use or test the boundaries of science, (3) doctors may be impatient, not taking the time to educate and empower patients, (4) doctors do not feel it is their responsibility to tell you every detail or secret for success, and (5) they may not know some secrets that can benefit you.

Your knowledge may cause a disruption to a system in place. His training and approach may be different from your ideas and his ego and expertise may be challenged if you know something he doesn't. Besides, business is threatened if you discover you do not need him, his drugs or his technology.

(1) HOW TO AVOID AN EPISIOTOMY

An episiotomy is a surgical cut in the perineum to enlarge the vagina. This unkind and painful cut was done to over 30% of first time mothers in the 1980's (Episiotomy rates vary among doctors), and has decreased to approximately 10%. Some doctors prefer to perform an episiotomy rather than risk a possible tear.

Here's how you can avoid an episiotomy:

1. Do Kegel exercises. Pelvic muscles should be exercised during pregnancy and throughout your lifetime to augment good women's health. Strong muscles are useful for delivery and help increase sexual peak experiences. Don't forget to do them immediately following birth.
2. Have your husband perform "perineal massage" during the last 6-8 weeks of pregnancy. This will help strengthen the muscles for delivery.
3. Do squatting and tailor-sitting exercises during pregnancy.
4. Have your birth attendant apply warm compresses on the perineum during birth.
5. Deliver the baby in a standing, squatting or kneeling position. This helps to prevent against tearing by up to 10%.
6. Do not hurry the birth or be overly aggressive about pushing.

7. Tell your doctor you do not want an episiotomy. Let him know that you are planning to do everything possible to ensure that your body will be ready to give birth and that you do not want to be a "routine" case.

(2) HOW TO AVOID A C-SECTION

Modern inventions allow us to lead busier and more complicated lives. Most of us are hurried with our activities and responsibilities. We seek to control our chaotic lives by scheduling and planning. The prevalence of C-sections is an outgrowth of our hurriedness and need for predictability. There are valid reasons for C-sections, but many C-sections are done for convenience and not as a last resort. Remember C-sections are major surgery. Researchers estimate that the true need for C-sections is around 5% of all deliveries. Approximately 33% (depending on the doctor and hospital) of women end up with a C-section. Failure to progress, a large baby, baby's heart rate stopped or baby in distress are common reasons for C-sections.

Here's how you can avoid a C-section:

1. Make it a goal of your pregnancy and birth to deliver vaginally. Prepare mentally, physically and be persistent with your doctor.
2. Arrive at the hospital well into labor. Once you are there, you will have to deliver within a certain time period, whether the baby is ready or not. Medical professionals are somewhat impatient. C-sections are sometimes performed because the doctor is in distress; he has a failure to wait or wants to avoid litigation if something should go wrong with a vaginal birth. C-sections are more risky than vaginal births. There is a higher chance of infection and other risks to the baby and mother.
3. Take a Bradley childbirth class during pregnancy.

4. Don't take drugs during labor. Epidurals may dull the pain, but they dull your ability to be fully involved and often lead to further intervention. Statistics vary, but it is estimated that epidural use increases a chance of a C-section by 35%.

(3) INCONCLUSIVE TESTS AND TECHNOLOGY

Many patients put a lot of credibility in test results and technological revelations. You need to know that (1) test results are not 100% accurate (2) you may be faced with an abortion decision (or pressure) if the Alpha-fetoprotein (AFP) or amniocentesis tests reveal an abnormality and (3) the implementation of technology results in a medicalized birth. The more medicalized the birth, the less emotionally, physically, and spiritually involved you will be. Less involvement usually means less satisfaction.

Many women receive abnormal results on their AFP test and go on to deliver healthy, normal babies. Others abort their babies based on test results. Each couple will have to make their own decision. More and more women are choosing to forego the AFP test and amniocentesis since they will keep their babies regardless of a physical or mental handicap.

Most people do not realize that the American College of Obstetrics and Gynecology, the American College of Radiology and the U.S. Preventive Services Task Force all recommend AGAINST routine ultrasound screening of low-risk pregnancies.

C-section decisions are made when the EFM indicates that the baby is in distress. Studies assert that EFMs have attributed to a high C-section rate and there is no evidence that EFMs are beneficial for childbirth. They also restrict movement for the expectant mother.

(4) THE RISKS AND EFFECTS OF LEGAL DRUGS DURING LABOR

Drugs carry risks and are harmful to the unborn and newly born. "The Five Standards for Safe Childbearing" was a classical text I found useful in the 1990's. Now there are many other resources that discuss the risks of drugs that are used to ease the pains of birth. I will leave it up to you to research your concerns.

While the mother may receive an appropriate dose of medication, the effects may be magnified ten to twenty times in the unborn baby. Women are unaware of the potential toxic effects to the unborn and are often unaware that a developing newborn and child can be affected for up to four or more years from drugs used in the delivery room.

More than twenty-eight side effects of epidurals have been reported. Some of the long term effects to the mother include persistent backaches, postpartum feelings of loss or regret, bladder dysfunction, decreased perineal sensation and decreased sexual function. I don't know about you, but if you told me there was a chance of lifelong consequences in my sex life as a result of taking drugs in childbirth, there's no way I'd take any drugs just to help me get through an hour or two of pain.

Effects of epidurals on the baby include: fetal distress, abnormal fetal heartrate, jaundice, breastfeeding and bonding problems, and poor muscle strength. Many of these babies need neonatal intensive care and it is suspected that babies and children may show signs of hyperactivity for up to seven years. Some psychiatrists have even pondered if there is a correlation between a drugged birth and ADD, ADHD, ODD and other hyperactive disorders.

Women are willing to take chances with their unborn baby because they are not fully educated about risks. They place their comfort above the health of their baby. Some drugs used in childbirth may cause permanent damage in children. Psychiatrists have labeled a few disorders with causes stemming from traumatic births, which almost always occur at the hands of doctors who use an assortment of drugs during a surgical or heavily intervened birth.

Drugs dull the sensation of birth. Neither pain nor pleasure is experienced in its entirety. The loud and intense noise that laboring women often make during natural childbirth is misinterpreted or embarrassing to medical practitioners. In the absence of drugs, a mother nearing birth will often make noises comparable to orgasmic moans. The birth release is a combination of pain and pleasure, mostly pleasure during the final seconds of birth. Adults misinterpret this ecstasy as agony and seek to block a true, full expression by the laboring woman. The more often drugs are used during birth, the less likely women report peak birth experiences.

Helen Wessel and others attribute postpartum depression to the absence of a birth climax. Women who are not fully awake and aware cannot feel the release after the baby is born. "This climax is essential. A mother who has missed it and had a passive, frigid birth, due to anesthetics, local injections or hypnosis, still is emotionally in a state of expectancy. She looks at her child, but experiences no euphoria, no sense of exhilaration." (Sousa 1976: 88)

"Biologically, our bodies want to finish labor and give birth triumphantly, with our senses intact...One researcher has found that the mother's endorphin level after a cesarean birth is lower than after the exertion of an unmedicated, vaginal birth." (Korte 1990: 37)

Here's a common scenario found in hospitals across the country: Pitocin used to speed up labor often leads to strong contractions and women find themselves requesting an epidural. Epidurals require continuous fetal monitoring which is restrictive and uncomfortable for the patient. In order to push, a woman needs to focus mentally at the moment she feels physical sensations. But epidurals dull the pain and seem to cloud the mind and body from this most important task. So the epidural detracts from the ability to push and sometimes leads to a C-section, which would have been totally unnecessary had drugs been avoided.

Studies show that C-sections present at least three to five times greater risk of death to the mother than vaginal delivery and an increased rate of complications in subsequent pregnancies.

It is assumed that women want to escape rather than cope with pain and fear. There is little discussion by doctors about fear; there doesn't need to be with the drugs and interventions that are used during labor and delivery.

Avoid drugs during labor and delivery because: (1) they are unsafe (2) they interfere with the brain-body chemistry before, during and after birth (3) they affect immediate breastfeeding success (4) they decrease the likelihood of a pleasurable birth release (5) they affect the alertness and energy level of the mother and baby, and (6) they affect postpartum attachment and bonding.

(5) HIS GOALS AND YOUR GOALS ARE DIFFERENT

There is an assumption that patients are not medically interested or knowledgeable and that they want to do whatever it takes to avoid pain. No one wants pain, but the main objective of birth should not be to avoid pain. Doctor-managed birth, overuse of technology, adherence to medical dogmas, and reliance on tests detract from the specialness of pregnancy and birth. Patients are not encouraged to take responsibility for themselves, because if they did, they would not need the establishment. Submission to authority is expected and the authority sometimes abuses its power, both intentionally and unintentionally.

OPTIMIST MEETS PESSIMIST. The first thing many healthy pregnant women do is seek a doctor's care. The patient arrives upbeat and enthusiastic while the doctor is looking for a problem to diagnose. The medical system supports the doctor's philosophy. "..Medical institutions, medical drug manufacturers, medical device industries, and medical professionals, in general, receive their benefits and their incomes in an amount proportional to the abundance of abnormality, sickness and complications." (Stewart 1997: 23) Over the course of several months, a doctor's borderline pessimism can replace the patient's optimism to the extent that she is monitoring herself for problems.

PROTECTOR VERSUS ENCOURAGER. Many doctors want to protect laboring women from physical and emotional harm. Problems arise when the protector does not fully understand the needs of who he is protecting. Many doctors do not personally know their patients. The protector's perceptions, beliefs and external constraints contribute to his treatment of what he believes to be the problem. While focusing on the solution, doctors miss the opportunity to act as encouragers. Laboring women are vulnerable and need encouragement.

WANT VERSUS NEED. Women want to have a baby and while medical professionals want to help them by being useful. Women go to a doctor to get what is needed and if nothing is needed, the doctor may discover a situation that requires his expertise. "That many women feel they have failed in one way or another in their births is not due to the method they practice but to the expectation of failure built into every hospital staff. It is this patronizing, negative attitude - more than the technology that spawns it - that makes natural childbirth a deception in the modern hospital. If women were to succeed at having their babies spontaneously and in an uncomplicated fashion, requiring only assistance and not intervention, then the hospital staff, trained in crisis and disease, would find itself with nothing medically to do." (Arms 1975:142) Almost fifty years later, this observation still rings true.

MATTER OVER MIND. Doctors focus on the physical elements of birth, excluding the psychological and emotional aspects, which impact couples more profoundly and for a longer period of time than the physical event. Psychological caretaking is not a function of an obstetrician; they do not attach much significance to mental attitude and imagery for a successful pregnancy and birth. A doctor who treats the woman as "matter" rather than a "mind" relies on drugs, tools and technology.

FINANCIAL INCENTIVES. The doctor's goal is to provide a valuable service and to make a profit while avoiding lawsuits. Doctors are more apt to submit to insurance company requirements than patients' desires. Patients should remember that the delivery of their baby is part of a business. They should not be surprised when they are not able to choose the hospital or doctor as they go into labor and prepare for delivery.

Whether they operate a private practice or work for an organization, obstetricians are part of a business ($34 billion in 2005 and $50 billion in 2013, for approximately four million births). Their goal is to make profits and avoid lawsuits. Lucrative profits can be made as more man-made assistance is provided for women in the childbearing years (and beyond): epidurals, C-sections, routine tests, ultrasounds, surgeries, procedures, prescriptions, artificial contraceptives; fertility drugs and menopausal hormone treatment plans.

The question I want you to ask of your health care provider is: "Is this absolutely, medically necessary, in my case?"

In 2013, the average cost for prenatal care, a vaginal birth in a hospital and basic newborn care was $30,000. For a C-section, the average cost was $50,000. Twenty years ago, many insurance coverage plans paid for most of the childbirth expenses. Today, new parents can expect to pay an average of $4,000 out of pocket for prenatal care and a hospital birth attended by a doctor.

(6) BIRTH IS AN UNCOMPLICATED PROCESS

Physiologically, birth is a straightforward process. Human females can expect a forty-week gestation period. Fetal development and the process of labor and delivery are universal. Birth becomes unnatural when we interfere with the process and make demands on a baby that isn't ready to be born. Technology can save lives and assist high-risk deliveries, but it often complicates perfectly normal births. Women are persuaded to take drugs and forced to endure internal exams and continuous monitoring. Patients who realize that birth is a simple biological function may one day decide to not subject themselves to obstetrics, which can complicate pregnancy and birth.

(7) YOUR DOCTOR MAY NOT BE AN EXPERT IN NATURAL BIRTH

Traditional medicine emphasizes treatment for illness and abnormality. Obstetricians are surgeon-specialists. Medical school trains doctors to perform medical deliveries and few doctors gain experience or expertise in natural, vaginal deliveries. Obstetricians handle a greater number of healthy, routine pregnancies compared to high-risk cases. In order to make themselves (and technology) useful, some doctors encourage the use of drugs during birth. This is what they know, what they've been trained for and what they value. What could be a satisfying, natural birth for many women often turns into a "high-tech" delivery.

Doctors who deal exclusively with high-risk pregnancies may be prone to considering birth as unsafe, abnormal and something women should fear. Pregnant women should be cautious when dealing with doctors who believe that childbirth is dangerous.

Women's health professionals offer surgery, chemical dependence and intervention. If it cannot be prescribed, cut or tampered with to facilitate a quick outcome, there may not be much incentive to help patients. It has been my experience and many others that the medical employees do not wait on minor problems or a process that might take a lot of time to unfold. They do not wean women from chemical dependence or encourage healthier solutions. They are trained to use drugs and procedures.

Women who want to have a natural birth need to be extremely persistent within the traditional medical system or seek alternatives to hospital deliveries.

(8) YOU ARE NOT IN CONTROL OF YOUR OWN BIRTH

It is difficult to feel in control of your situation upon entering a hospital. Paperwork must be completed; rules and regulations must be followed. It becomes a battle for an individualized, as opposed to institutionalized, birth. The birthing Mom may feel defensive in order to ensure she gets what she wants. Hospitals are brightly lighted, non-private, ungentle environments. Many women conclude that they do not have to act tough (and avoid drugs) for some idealistic notion (an unmedicated vaginal delivery).

Rather than trusting nature, women seek to control and manipulate it. A special and satisfying birth requires the release of any inhibitions. Expectant women who acknowledge that there is a moment of intense vulnerability during childbirth can more easily resign themselves to the experience. You are not in control during the natural onset of labor, nor are you in control when your doctor decides to induce labor or perform a C-section. But you can control your thoughts and beliefs about pregnancy and delivery.

Your birth attendant's beliefs affect your birth. You may want to present a birth plan* to your doctor, but you must be assertive when you give birth. Remember that you are paying your doctor to make decisions, some of which you may not like.

Every day, unsuspecting mothers are violated in the delivery room. Pitocin is used to speed up birth; abdomens are aggressively manipulated to extract the placenta. Women are induced only to deliver a premature baby who needs special care. C-sections are performed more frequently than is medically necessary. Women are hooked up to monitors, given IVs and forced to give birth in an uncomfortable position. Expectant mothers are given drugs to alleviate pain and those drugs silence them. Ultimately, women are not encouraged, shown or taught how to give birth successfully.

Part III contains chapters which describe specific ways you can take back some control over your birth.

(9) YOUR MENTAL OUTLOOK IS VERY IMPORTANT

Your greatest hidden treasure is your attitude. You can choose acceptance, frustration, resignation or many other perspectives during your birth event, regardless of where it is, when it takes place or who is present. Your attitude, intentions, and perseverance have a MAJOR effect on the birth as well as other events in your life. Those who are extremely fearful tend to approach pregnancy and childbirth timidly.

"There seems to be a relation between anxiety, overt or covert, and the length of labor. Uterine dysfunction may also be associated with concealed anxiety. Harry Bakow found that mothers who were anxious during pregnancy and who expressed more concern over the course of their pregnancy more often had babies who got into distress at delivery. Recent studies suggest that women likely to have complications during childbirth are those who during pregnancy manifested a negative attitude to the pregnancy, showed concern for the condition of the child, saw their employment as being disrupted, listed a greater number of contacts with women who had complicated pregnancies, and described their own mother's health as poor." (Macfarlane 1976: 18)

In "Visualizations for an Easier Childbirth," Carl Jones poses five questions a woman should ask herself before choosing a place to give birth: "(1) Am I the center of my childbearing experience in this place? (2) Am I fully in charge? (3) Is this the place where I want to begin a new family? (4) Is this the best place to make the transition to life outside the womb? (5) Do I receive the emotional support I deserve in this place?" (Jones 1988: 42) Arriving at honest answers to these questions increases the likelihood of a positive mental outlook in order to have a rewarding birth event.

(10) HOW TO HAVE A SUCCESSFUL BIRTH EXPERIENCE

DURING YOUR PREGNANCY: Set goals and be persistent with your birth attendant. Avoid unnecessary or risky tests. Avoid ultrasounds, unless absolutely, medically necessary. Please investigate current research that shows the risks of ultrasound. Distance yourself from negative or fear-inducing people. Your pregnancy and birth are part of a dream you are fulfilling; do not let anyone try to steal your dream. Make a plan for birth. Take a Bradley childbirth class. Find a doula or labor coach to attend your birth. Involve your spouse. Follow proper nutrition. Prepare mentally, spiritually and physically.

DURING YOUR BIRTH: Keep up your energy by drinking and eating throughout labor. Arrive at the hospital or go into the delivery room well into labor. Be confident. Maintain an upright position during labor and birth. Avoid the electronic fetal monitor, internal fetal monitor and drugs. Visualize the baby's passage into the world rather than focusing on your pain. And finally, try to keep your birth as quiet, comfortable and stress-free as possible. Successful birthing depends on concentration, alertness and confidence.

*birth plan - detailed instructions presented to your doctor and hospital staff outlining your intentions for birth.

HELPFUL RESOURCES:

Davis-Floyd, Robbie. "Birth as an American Rite of Passage." 1992. Univ. of California Press, Berkeley, CA.

Griesemer, Lynn M. "Unassisted Homebirth: An Act of Love." 1998. Terra Publishing, Tampa, FL.

Jones, Carl. "Mind Over Labor: A Breakthrough Guide to Giving Birth." 1988, Penguin Books, Inc. NY, NY.

Mendelsohn, Robert, M.D. "Confessions of a Medical Heretic." 1979. Warner Books, Chicago, Ill.

_____. "Male Practice: How Doctors Manipulate Women." 1982. Contemporary
Books, Inc. Chicago, Ill.

Moran, Marilyn A. "Pleasurable Husband / Wife Childbirth: The Real Consummation of Married Love." 1997. Terra Publishing, Tampa, FL (out of print).

Sears, Martha, R.N. and William, M.D. "The Birth Book: Everything You Need to Know to have a Safe and Satisfying Birth." 1994. Little Brown & Co., Boston, MA.

REFERENCES CITED:

Arms, Suzanne. "Immaculate Deception: A New Look at Women and Childbirth in America." 1975. Houghton Mifflin, Co., Boston, MA.

Jones, Carl. "Visualizations for an Easier Childbirth." 1988. Simon & Schuster, NY, NY.

Korte, Diana and Scaer, Roberta. "A Good Birth, A Safe Birth." 1990. Bantam, NY, NY.

Macfarlane, Aidan. "The Psychology of Childbirth." 1977, Harvard University Press, Cambridge, MA.

Sousa, Marion. "Childbirth at Home." 1976. Prentice-Hall Inc., Englewood Cliffs, NJ.

Stewart, David, Ph.D. "The Five Standards for Safe Childbearing." 1997. NAPSAC International, Marble Hill, MO.

CHAPTER 4: EXPLOITATION AT BIRTH

Many aspects of modern birth are exploitative to couples. Expectant couples, for the most part, are unaware of the exploitations. Since many people fear pain and the act of birth, they place complete faith in the medical system to help them make it through their ordeal. Couples willingly conform to the medical directives during pregnancy and birth, directives that are not always in the best interests of their safety and comfort.

Women are put in subservient roles when they contract services from a doctor. The doctor makes the final decisions and is the manager of the birth. Exploitations can occur if the medical professional's loyalty is aligned with the hospital and insurance companies rather than the patient. Monetary goals and professional or community reputation matter. At the same time, many Americans are not concerned with an emotionally empowering birth because they are preoccupied with the myth that birth is unsafe and dangerous.

When birth is treated as a medical event, the body is the focus. When doctors orchestrate the birth event, the father is robbed of the opportunity to touch his wife in passionate or sexual ways that would soothe her discomforts and provide encouragement. Some couples avoid holding hands, kissing or expressing private gestures since they are in a public setting. During a few of my hospital births, my husband admitted that he held back tears of joy after the births.

If you view birth as a sexual event, then it seems logical that a certain amount of foreplay can take place during labor. Homebirthers have shared some of their foreplay secrets that have made for a more loving birth, shorter labor, less pain and more pleasure (emotionally and physically). Here are a few: (1) nipple stimulation releases oxytocin and often triggers contractions (2) semen released into a woman's body stimulates the release of Relaxin which softens and opens up the cervix (3) perineum massage after 36 weeks gestation can eliminate the need for an episiotomy, and (4) applying warm washcloths to the perineum right before birth can be very soothing.

There is no foreplay in hospitals. Medications replace sex play. Pitocin is the synthetic replacement for natural oxytocin; prostaglandin gel used to soften the cervix is actually pig semen; and episiotomies are painful and unkind cuts made to the perineum in order to enlarge the opening for the passage of the baby.

As mentioned earlier, we may be setting ourselves up for exploitations if we submit, conform or relinquish power. Our assumptions and perceptions, fears, or lack of goals can also leave us vulnerable. Women who want to avoid a "high tech" pregnancy often are not bold enough to say no. Instead of avoiding all of the routine testing to confirm that the baby will be "perfect," they go along with the unnecessary blood tests, ultrasounds, amniocentesis and other procedures that "science" insists upon.

The childbirth business exceeds $50 billion dollars a year; we have excellent technology; men and women are smarter than ever; yet the U.S. ranked 34th in the world in maternal and neonatal safety up until 2007 and now ranks 61st out of 179 countries in maternal safety. The rate of infant death has gone from 12 babies per 100,000 mothers in 1990 to 28 / 100,000 in 2013. It more than doubled! All the new and improved decorating in the hospital maternity wards has not made for safer births.

Protocol in the delivery room is disrespectful to some degree. Women are told to lie on a table disguised as a bed, monitored by equipment, and given internal exams which can be painful. The staff comes and goes freely; women are persuaded to take drugs to ease their pain; and they are told when to push. Shorter, successful labor and delivery depends upon women reacting to their bodily cues, not outsiders deciding what should happen next.

Women need silence to concentrate on the enormous task at hand. Many animals are treated better at birth than humans. Can you imagine the medical system intruding upon cats? Inductions and C-sections for 33% of the cat population? Tests, monitors, episiotomies, vacuum extractors? How is it that animals are birthing more perfectly than humans?

I cannot offer quick solutions to avoiding exploitations at birth. Expectant mothers must decide what they are willing to settle for and start from there. There are many gentle and kind employees who are doing their best to ensure a dignified hospital birth experience, but there are dozens of exploitations that take place every day in delivery rooms around the world. The first step is regaining personal control and responsibility.

PART II: NEW PERSPECTIVES ON BIRTH

CHAPTER 5: DOCTOR-DELIVERED BABIES AND NATURAL LAW: A CONFLICT BETWEEN THE TWO

The following article was written by Marilyn A. Moran.

Dr. William Hazlett, an obstetrician in Kingston, PA, was one of the pioneers in the 1960's to allow husbands to accompany their wives into the delivery room when they were giving birth instead of sitting in the fathers' waiting room until the birth was over. Furthermore, he encouraged them to 'catch' their own babies while he sat in a corner making suggestions. It was his feeling that the self-esteem of husband and wife was heightened when they actively gave birth together.

In a 1967 article entitled "The Male Factor in Obstetrics," Hazlett had some sharp words for his fellow obstetricians. He spoke of the

"danger...in obstetrical technology's intimacy with the woman's procreative function and its ability and robot compulsion to subvert that function, given the chance, to its own end which...is the apotheosis of the obstetrician. Not only apotheosis toward which obstetrical technology drives him, but also androgynization to which the obstetrician rises...When he gives birth operatively, he symbolically conquers the woman. More than that, however, he incorporates femaleness. Thus he becomes, artificially, the androgyne, that union of male and female principles which according to legend and myth we all have lost, according to philosophers, theologians and psychologists we all as incomplete persons aspire to. If intuitively we do want to return, rising higher to a spiritual androgyny, it is not for me to say that technology cannot or will not take us there. Nor should I say that the obstetrician ought not strive for it. But it is evil when he uses the woman as a means to an end."

It was refreshing to rediscover these words of Hazlett's. I have long wrestled with the propriety of what obstetricians do in assisting a woman to give birth. I came to the conclusion that their actions are highly inappropriate and thought I had come up with a novel idea. But Hazlett beat me to it all the while. It was probably he, moreover, who planted the idea in my mind decades ago when I first read the article.

My first seven babies were medicated 'deliveries' where I was knocked out hours before the birth and sometimes didn't wake up until hours later. I thought it was a wonderful way to give birth. I knew nothing, saw nothing, and felt nothing except the stitches which I felt for weeks afterward.

Then in 1966 I had my first Lamaze birth where I was awake and aware. What a difference that was. My doctor wouldn't let my husband in the delivery room. But he was in the delivery room three years later for the birth of my second Lamaze baby. Reflecting afterwards on my sensations and emotions during those two births I realized that birth is not something a person does in front of strangers. It is too personal and private a thing. So when the next (our last) child was born I deliberately stayed home and gave birth to him with just my husband with me in the seclusion of our bedroom. It was truly marvelous!

For 14 years I published a newsletter for do-it-yourself homebirth couples called "The New Nativity." In it I printed 244 personal accounts written by couples who did what we did. While each experience was different from the others, all were very beautiful and extremely rewarding for the couples involved.

Many of the women in their birth accounts mentioned that they, too, had reservations about what their obstetricians had done during the births of their previous children. Jayne Meyer wrote, "We always questioned why people put more faith in the doctor than in God. We were both raised with strong moral virtues and I always felt dirty with a male OB. I could never understand why, if someone had four more years of school than I, they were allowed to monkey with something I had worked 21 years to keep chaste for only my husband."

Another mother, Jennifer Gordon, wrote, "Giving birth is such an intimate affair, it should be kept private. I always said the doctor wasn't there when I conceived, so why should he be there at the birth? Besides, I don't want any man looking between my legs. I don't care if that man sees 50 vaginas a day! As a matter of fact, I didn't seek a doctor's services at all during this last pregnancy." Neither did she go to a doctor for the next three pregnancies which each resulted in an intimate husband/wife love encounter homebirth.

At about the same time that "The New Nativity" was being published, statements calling birth a sexual experience were suddenly appearing in books and articles. Christopher Derrick, George Gilder, Sheila Kitzinger, Helen Wessel, Lewis E. Mehl, M.D., Michel Odent, M.D., Thomas Verny, M.D., Lonnie Barbach, Ph.D., Barbara Rothman, plus many others spoke of it as such. It's no wonder the homebirth mothers were critical of what had been done to them previously by obstetricians!

Birth is, indeed, a sexual experience. It is as much a part of the conjugal communion between husband and wife as is the act of coitus. This time the roles of male and female are simply reversed. It is the wife who now has a significant, tangible love gift to present to her beloved spouse, one he has been silently longing to receive during the 40 weeks of pregnancy. As she personally and deliberately eases her love gift, the baby, from her body directly into the organ of her husband's cupped hands their nuptial experience is brought to a close just as surely as the offering of Jesus on the cross to his Heavenly Father with the words, "Into thy hands I commend my spirit," brought to a close the biphasic act of Redemption. In both instances the "holy exchange of gifts" was required. Nothing less would suffice.

Now let us examine the morality of what has traditionally transpired in hospital delivery rooms. As we have seen, one obstetrician used the word evil in regard to what doctors do there. Is it evil of obstetricians to come between men and their wives during the sexual act of birth? An appeal to natural law should help clarify this issue.

According to the late Catholic theologian John Courtney Murray, S.J., natural law theory had only one threefold presupposition: "that man is intelligent, that reality is intelligible, and that it be obeyed in its demands for action or abstention."

There is no mystery why couples would want to give birth in an intimate, husband/wife way. It is a sexual experience and, therefore, an inherent part of their sacramental vow to serve the needs of each other, all of them. As to how they go about it, that too is answered by the statement that it is a sexual experience.

The birthing couple has many faculties for carrying out the task at hand which, customarily, they have been constrained from using. One is deep, warm kisses. If the mother's face and mouth are relaxed the other end of her anatomy will be, too, permitting the descent of the baby. Mary Finocchario wrote in her homebirth account, "Lou gave me one of his long Italian kisses and within seconds the baby door flew open." Nipple stimulation works wonders, too. Researchers have found that it causes the posterior lobe of the pituitary to release the hormone oxytocin which contracts the uterus. This helps expel the baby and also prevents unnecessary blood loss following birth. Finally, there is the hormone Relaxin. It softens the cervix of the uterus and also lengthens pelvic ligaments, both of which are important preparations for the gentle birth of the baby. Although its existence and function have been known since 1927, it wasn't until 1982 that researchers discovered it in human seminal plasma, at "high levels," no less, per Dr. Gillian Bryant-Greenwood of the Department of Anatomy and Reproductive Biology, at the University of Hawaii. Thus, when a couple has coitus during labor the husband is able to provide his wife with the precise hormone that she needs for the safe and gentle birth of their child.

The above-mentioned faculties were given to humanity by what the Baltimore Catechism called our "all-knowing, all-loving, all-provident" Creator at the dawn of time. They were put there to be used. While it is possible to be technologically "delivered" without them, as Dr. Joseph Warshaw of Yale Medical School said regarding premature infants kept alive for weeks and months in incubators, "Mother Nature does it better. A lot of what we do is trying to catch up."

The reality of childbirth is that there is little to worry about if the provisions of nature, or God as I prefer to say, are put to use. What technology can provide is strictly second-rate. This goes for the delivery room as well as the neonatal intensive care unit. Smart people don't scorn the natural in favor of the technological.

As we have seen, when couples are told the truth about birth and are encouraged to think about it and to talk it over between themselves, the thought of a hospital "delivery" becomes increasingly repulsive to them. Deep down inside, both husbands and wives know that giving birth is something which is best done by themselves in the privacy of their own bedrooms. Many couples, upon discovering this childbirth choice, immediately opt for it because they intuitively know it's the right thing to do. Others have to give it some thought before they become determined enough to defy culture and give birth in an intimate, love encounter way instead. One mother reported, after giving birth alone with her husband, "My only regret is that I did not do it 10 years ago when my husband first wanted to try it!"

Another couple planned to give birth at home with the help of a midwife. But as they searched for the perfect attendant, the mother realized that "each midwife seemed like she was taking over and I very much wanted to share this act with my husband. After thinking over the do-it-yourself option, we knew in our hearts and minds that this was the way to go."

One man called the idea "captivating." Another, in his 60s, who had been with his wife in the delivery room each of the seven times that she gave birth, said, "I never had the terrific experience of her delivering the baby into my hands! That must be something." It is tragic that he and his wife were needlessly denied the chance to experience this exquisitely marvelous "something."

Birth has been bowdlerized to the great detriment of couples. We must reach out to them with the truth about the conjugal act of birth. Until we do, they will continue to be robbed of an important marital love act.

Thus we have a natural law argument against hospital deliveries, the syllogism for which would be:

(1) It is wrong to rob a married couple of the opportunity to express their love in an intimate, marital act.

(2) The delivery of a baby by technologists in the hospital robs a married couple of the opportunity to express their love in the intimate, marital act of childbirth.

(3) Therefore, the delivery of a baby by technologists in the hospital is wrong.

By examining the human body and how it works a functional design to the organs becomes apparent. That's one of the reasons why there is a growing movement today to abandon the practice of circumcising baby boys. Activists say that the foreskin of the penis serves a purpose and it should not be disdainfully sacrificed. Kenneth Purvis, M.D., wrote,

"Has the supreme being made a minor blunder in his blueprint for the male of the species?"

Judging by the near-universal custom in this country of hospital deliveries of babies by high-tech professionals, it would seem that God has made a major blunder for the female of the species as well. However, upon studying the effect of marital intimacies on the progress of labor it becomes readily apparent that it is we, ourselves, who have made a big mistake and not our Maker.

There is something else about hospital deliveries that is bizarre. Because forceps can damage both baby and mother, the use of a vacuum extractor during birth is gaining in popularity. One report says it consists of a suction cup being inserted, "by well-trained individuals," into the mother's vagina. "The cup fits on the baby's head, and a vacuum pump firmly fixes it there. The doctor or birthing assistant gently pulls to draw the infant out. It sounds strange, but it has been proved quite effective."

It would probably be effective, also, for a husband to have a suction cup attached to the tip of his penis to allow someone to gently draw out seminal fluid. But, as the Church has repeatedly stated, such action would be contrary to natural law.

We have a double standard here. If such behavior is nonsensical (and sinful) for a husband, it must be just as much so for a wife. Both violate nature because both separate the unitive from the procreative aspects of sexual love.

Therefore, another natural law argument against hospital deliveries could be stated with the following syllogism:

(1) All genital expressions belong within the framework of intimate, husband/wife relations, exclusively.

(2) Birth is a genital expression.

(3) Therefore, birth belongs within the framework of intimate, husband/wife relations, exclusively.

So far we have covered two of the three sections of natural law mentioned by Father John Courtney Murray as it pertains to the birth of babies. The reality is that there are simple lovemaking techniques readily available to birthing couples which permit them to give birth by themselves. As we have seen from the many anecdotes mentioned above, when couples hear about this 'method' of birthing and give it careful thought, with rare exceptions they choose to give birth this way. It just seems right to them in contrast to the medical model of birth.

While the couples who give birth at home in an intimate husband/wife way do use their innate intelligence, that can't be said about those who mindlessly go to the hospital delivery route. Donald DeMarco in his book, "Biotechnology and the Assault on Parenthood," referred to "Humanae Vitae," by Pope Paul VI, in which contraception was called, "an intrinsically disordered human act" because it separated the unitive from the procreative aspects of human sexuality. The same goes for "in-vitro" fertilization, the freezing of human embryos, and the implantation of fertilized eggs into third-party surrogates. Professor Charles Rice, of Notre Dame Law School, in his review of the DeMarco book called them "the idiocies of technological parenthood."

What about vacuum extractors to pull babies out of mothers' bodies, electrodes screwed into babies' scalps while still "in utero," and delivery tables to which mothers' legs and wrists are strapped, immobilizing them? Aren't they "idiocies of technological parenthood," too?

Wasn't I an idiot to be drugged senseless for the births of my first seven babies?

Aren't hospital deliveries also "intrinsically disordered acts" because they, too, separate the unitive and procreative aspects of human sexuality?

As for man being intelligent, if even 50 really intelligent people had read and pondered Hazlett's article when "Child and Family" published it in its Fall 1967 issue, there'd be no "in-vitro" fertilization, surrogate mothers, or 1.5 million abortions a year in the U.S. today. Our young people, instead of being in the dark, would know that the sexual experience of birth is an integral part of the covenant of marriage. Therefore, they'd postpone engaging in sexual activity until they could do it right, from start to finish. Babies would be born at home in a private, loving, husband/wife way, with two parents to love and provide for them instead of with only one as is the case all too often today. And the word Catholic would be removed from all hospitals where obstetricians continue to ply their unholy trade.

To decline to give adequate attention to the conjugal act of birth because of squeamishness is not an intelligent thing to do. It's immature and unbecoming one baptized into the life of Christ.

Professor Janet Smith writes, "Man does not act in accord with reason {that is, he violates the natural law; he does what is immoral} when he opposes the design of God." It is the design of God that the birthing woman get nipple stimulation from her husband during labor because this action provides her with a hormone which will cause her uterus to contract. Doctors prefer to attach mother to an IV to administer Pitocin, a synthetic substitute for oxytocin, and generally do so.

It is the design of God that the mother have coitus with her husband during labor so that the hormone Relaxin contained in his seminal plasma could alter her pelvis to permit the gentle descent of the baby without injury to its head. Doctors are experimenting with carbowax pessaries containing purified porcine Relaxin (from pigs) which are inserted into the vagina against the cervix in an effort to do the same thing.

It is the design of God that the birthing mother have perineal massage from her spouse, which keeps the tissues soft and elastic, to prevent the area from tearing during the birth process. Doctors prefer to do an episiotomy, a small cut to enlarge the opening of the vagina. Dr. Roy V. Boedecker, a St. Louis obstetrician, in extolling the episiotomy, said, "We inject a little Novocain, make a little cut, lift the baby out gently with forceps, then repair and restore the pelvic floor even better than God made it."

Obstetricians have made a mockery of the design of God regarding the sexual act of birth. Most married couples have gone along with their doctors' advice, thinking they had no choice. However, others have discovered there is a choice which simply entails loving as Christ loved, calmly, fearlessly, with no holding back, just resolutely doing what has to be done – and enjoying it!

Using the innate potential within themselves they are driving back the primordial darkness surrounding the sexual act of birth by enkindling the fire of love. May it never be allowed to go out.

"With three things I am delighted, for they are pleasing to the Lord and to men: Harmony among brethren, friendship among neighbors, and the mutual love of husband and wife." – Sirach 25:1

(Marilyn A. Moran is author of "Birth and the Dialogue of Love," "Happy Birth Days" and "Pleasurable Husband / Wife Childbirth: The Real Consummation of Married Love.")

CHAPTER 6: CHILDBIRTH: A FEMINIST ISSUE?

The most significant event in a woman's life - childbirth - has been largely ignored by the feminists. Well known feminists are silent about childbirth, which will be experienced by a majority of women at some point in their lives. When it comes to reproduction, feminists are more concerned with the right to choose abortion and artificial contraception.

Feminism emerges in at least three different forms. Radical feminists blame men for female inequality and believe that the oppression of women is fostered by marriage, motherhood, or any situation where women are "dependent" upon men. Social feminists view the economic class system as the problem and equate a woman's worth with the amount of her paycheck. Women's rights feminists strongly believe that people are created equal and deserve equal opportunity.

Because the feminist leadership seems to be dominated by radical and social feminists, you can see why childbirth is not important to them. Many feminists view babies as an interference with the pursuit of economic and career success.

Feminists are often reactive rather than proactive, reacting to the perceived threat of a woman's rights being taken away, as opposed to seeking fulfillment. This is understandable in a patriarchal culture. Traditional childbirth (obstetrician directed hospital delivery) is often exploitative to women and leaves little room for empowerment and fulfillment during a major, life-changing event.

INEQUITY

When we contract services with an obstetrician or midwife, we put ourselves in a subservient role. The expert has the ultimate power in childbirth since he or she will be the one to make major decisions in an emergency. Birth is based on someone else's philosophies and goals. A woman who has hired a doctor must remember that physicians control labor and conduct delivery. The burden is on the patient to assert her desires.

Since we do not have the ultimate power in these birth situations, we do not have full participation in our experiences and outcomes. We risk feeling dissatisfied, incomplete and regretful. The many women who leave the hospital after a satisfying birth experience will later wonder why they cannot identify the source of their discontent or why they are suffering from postpartum depression. The reason for this is that they had established what they thought was an equal partnership with their doctor. They were mistaken. The pregnancy has come to an end and they cling to the belief that there was an equal partnership, rather than a business relationship.

Birth is a choice. Women need to consider what they want for their birth and set goals. They need less harassment and judgment from others. Until childbirth is acknowledged as an issue worthy of attention and until women demand more from their caregivers, inequities will exist.

FAITH IN EXPERTS

As long as we continue to use their services, doctors perceive that their expertise is wanted and needed. They encourage us to patronize their businesses. We may feel as if we benefit from their services, but we will never be truly free unless we take charge by becoming our own experts. Whether we choose to employ doctors or birth at home, the key to good health is personal knowledge and action.

A biased view of childbirth is presented to us by movies, popular magazines, advertisers, hospitals and medical professionals. The medical profession has established itself as the legitimate authority on maternal and infant health, contraception, infertility, pregnancy, childbirth practices, postpartum management, infant feeding and childrearing. The public has eagerly accepted doctors as experts, without question. When we put all of our faith in others and disregard ourselves as an expert, we are often left feeling dependent, unconfident, inadequate, and afraid.

EXPLOITATION AND BONDAGE

When it comes to service, expect the best and you may get it; demand the best and you will get it. Many women do not expect much from their birth attendants or place they will give birth. It is not uncommon for several obstetricians to work for the same practice and couples to be surprised that the doctor of their choice does not deliver their baby. Until we set goals and become more assertive, we will be open to exploitation.

Since childbirth is a multi-billion dollar industry, it is no surprise that money is the motivation behind birth practices. Many doctors, pediatricians, hospitals and citizens would like to maintain current childbirth practices, especially when hundreds of jobs are at stake in every community. The profitability of the maternity section in some hospitals has become very important to the bottom line. It is not uncommon to see hospital advertisements luring patients into their place of business.

Feminists are adamant that "government does not belong in the bedroom making personal family decisions." However, midwife-attended homebirth is illegal in many states and feminists do not seem to be working hard to ensure greater opportunity and choice regarding birth. The medical establishment has been known to convince legislators of the "danger" and "inferiority" of midwifery and homebirths. How sad it is that the powerful monopoly wants to control and preside over birth choices.

Drugs given to alleviate pain silence women and are often harmful to them and their babies. Rather than rely on their instincts and comfort, patients must deliver a baby by conforming to rules, regulations and the hospital staff's convenience. Women are not encouraged, shown or taught how to give birth successfully.

Women's bodies are treated as machines, subject to painful internal examinations at the whim of the doctor and staff. Women are practically forced to give birth in an uncomfortable position on a table, while hooked up to an electronic fetal monitor or IV. Many are induced and go on to deliver premature babies who need special care.

Approximately 33% of babies born in the United States arrive via C-section, major surgery, which according to alternative birth advocates, should only occur in 5% of the pregnant population. As a comparison, 5% babies were born via C-section in 1970, 20% in 1996, and 30% in 2007. The rate is rising, not decreasing.

And how interesting that the World Health Organization (WHO) held firm to the "no more than 5%" C-section rate recommendation for decades. As of 2015, the WHO states that no more than 15% of births should be C-sections. It sounds less drastic to say that the USA's rate is doubled what it should be. Unless women's physiology has changed in the last decade or if there are some extreme reasons to increase the WHO's percentage, I would think that the 5% recommendation is the true representation of what should be happening as far as the need for C-sections.

WHAT WILL HAPPEN IF FEMINISTS CONTINUE TO IGNORE THE ISSUE OF CHILDBIRTH?

Feminists continue to disregard childbirth as a major women's issue as countless women submit to the current birth culture. Feminists have been concerned with women's rights, but if they are truly concerned with empowering women, they will realize that childbirth is an important rite of passage.

Feminists will become a more narrowly focused group if they do not expand their priorities to include issues which affect the majority of women, issues such as birth empowerment. Women are beginning to recognize the exploitation that currently abounds in traditional prenatal care and hospital deliveries. Feminists could be a pivotal force in raising awareness about birth practices in this country, if they cared.

CHAPTER 7: HOW INTIMATE BIRTH STRENGTHENS MARRIAGE

"No test has been sent you that does not come to all men. Besides, God keeps his promise. He will not let you be tested beyond your strength. Along with the test he will give you a way out of it so that you may be able to endure it." 1 Corinthians 10:13

On August 3, 1996, my husband and I gave birth to our fifth child. And on June 7, 2002, our son was born in the privacy of our bedroom. The births were very simple, natural events. The only difference was that we chose to have these babies at home, with no attendants - no doctor or midwife. Both children were born in the privacy of our bedroom - the same intimate setting as the conception. We were physically, mentally and spiritually prepared for the birth, yet many people considered this risky and radical behavior.

Those who obsess about what may go wrong jeopardize the opportunity to grow in deeper faith. When we invite God completely into our lives, the fear and worry dissipate. I am not implying that anyone who seeks medical attention or other people to help them solve their problems downplay the role of Christ in their lives. Certainly there are situations where medical attention is warranted.

But too often we lack confidence to confront the challenges of life or we delegate personal responsibility by seeking "experts." When we depend on ourselves, mediate initial excessive worry, and ask for God's assistance, we grow in faith, trust and confidence. Self-sufficiency during birth requires and results in an alert and empowered state of mind, qualities necessary for a successful, productive life.

The human body is perfectly designed and there is no reason why most births could not culminate in relatively effortless, natural births. Man has a way of treating his body abusively, from overeating, sexual promiscuity, alcohol and physical abuse to the more subtle abuses of fertility, pregnancy and childbirth: artificial contraception, extraneous medical testing and unnecessary (but economically profitable) medications, inductions and surgeries. For example, couples should consider that they may not only be maiming their bodies, but also their marriages when they consent to sterilization. Fully alive expression of sexuality leaves little room for intrusive barriers, including temporary and permanent interference with new life.

A majority of couples welcome children into their lives according to their own convenience and planning. So too, babies are delivered at everyone else's convenience but the baby's.

Any couple who has received the Sacrament of Matrimony might remember the phrase, "Let no man divide what God has joined together." Well, during childbirth, couples are unknowingly divided in the delivery room. The obstetrician takes center stage as the husband sits on the sideline. Fathers who travel through forty weeks of pregnancy knowing that they will be the first to touch and see their baby begin family life with a deep emotional attachment and commitment.

Unassisted homebirth, or birth in the absence of a midwife or obstetrician, offers many advantages over birth in an institutional setting, but there are several marital benefits of unassisted birth that are worth considering.

Mature love, strong marriages and satisfying birth experiences contribute to confidence in adulthood and a love for children. This leads to competent parenting and a rich, rewarding family life. Love involves a sharing of hopes and desires and the birth of a baby brings together the uniqueness of the couple.

Each partner wants his mate to be happy, healthy and successful. The other's needs are given a higher priority. Two people seem to merge and enhance each other's sense of aliveness. Partners must take the risk of giving all that they are and all that they have, of pouring themselves out completely, without reservations. Trust, respect and admiration blossom during an unassisted birth. True lovers are no longer two persons; they have achieved a unique identity together.

Marriage is mainly about unity and indissolubility, which is achieved through fidelity and mutual assistance. A" perfect" union requires spouses to mature, accept each other and reveal to each other new depths and facets of themselves. Faith, hope and trust are needed for love to reach a higher dimension. Conjugal love is enriched by trials, sufferings and sacrifices. Marriage is about the deepening of love.

People set themselves up for disappointment if they expect something extraordinary from their mates. It is not your mate's purpose to bring you happiness. Not even the perfect love relationship with a lifetime mate will bring complete satisfaction. People do not realize that they are seeking something outside themselves, a sense of spirituality or God. True joy occurs when there is a link between the flesh, the mind and the Divine, in the presence of lovers and God. This is possible during an unassisted homebirth.

Birth is able to unfold naturally and couples can be comfortable and uninhibited when there are no strangers making demands or other family members who bring their fears, expectations or subtle distractions. Because there is total privacy between lovers during an intimate birth, it is likely that there will be a fusion of personalities during the birth. Having a child is the most creative thing a couple can do and a baby is a permanent example of the joining of the couple's hearts and minds. If the parents share in the process of making and raising the child, they could have a meaningful sharing at the birth event.

Odds are against a couple trying to achieve a complete fusion in a situation where there are others present at the birth or if the setting is even somewhat uncomfortable. Intimate birth is so emotionally appealing that it's easy to lose sight of the physical pain that often accompanies childbirth. No separations between the couple, no small talk or interference from strangers, nobody giving commands or making demands - what a way to have a baby!

While the couple is strengthening their bond during the birth, they are also beginning parenthood with confidence. By seeing each other in a new situation that requires courage, a special, mutual respect takes place. If they triumph after a birth experience, they can do anything; they are ready to take on the world. Politicians, community and business leaders generally agree that the key to a strong society is strong families. What better place to strengthen marital harmony and family unity than with an unassisted homebirth?

CHAPTER 8: BIRTH FROM A RELIGIOUS PERSPECTIVE

As a practicing Catholic, I've thought a lot about unassisted birthing in the context of Catholicism. No theologian has written about it, so I assume that there is very little thought about a connection. "Theology of the Body," by John Paul II, revealed to me obvious connections to unassisted homebirth. In this chapter I want to present some new ideas to ponder. Many unassisted birthers are not Catholic and among Catholics, many are not drawn to unassisted birth. It is estimated that less than 1% of expectant mothers elect a homebirth and of that 1%, a small amount choose unassisted birth.

I can think of six or seven Catholics who have experienced unassisted homebirth and contacted me during the past twenty years, expressing a belief that there is a relationship between unassisted birth and Catholicism. I realize that this chapter may appeal to only a handful of people.

I want to begin this section by talking about marriage. The Catholic Church gives us the Sacrament of Matrimony. Many people do not realize how deep and beautiful this is and the graces that are available to us. The priest is a conduit through which Christ seals the couple's love during the Sacrament of Matrimony. It is an exclusive and permanent union in which the couple is also united to Christ. We give the gift of self to our partner and to God as we leave our old life behind and forge a new one – a life that is formed for the betterment of our souls, our sanctification and our salvation.

The desire for love is a universal human need. People want to love, but have a greater need to be loved, by God and others, whether it is within their immediate family, by a spouse, or friends. The truly holy person knows and experiences love – love of God and love of others. Some people make the mistake of seeking perfect love and happiness in another human being, and fail to consider that we are all imperfect and are not capable of a "perfect" love relationship. Perfect happiness is found in our infinite Creator, not a finite, fallible creature.

I would like to mention a few aspects of love. True love requires sacrifice. True love is rooted in charity and "agape" love – doing things for your partner that you may not want to do or that he or she can easily do, without your help. Tasks are freely done out of genuine, unconditional love for the person, without any expectation or anticipation of reward or praise.

Love involves the soul, not just the body. It demands a gift of self. It requires a decision and commitment, an orientation of the will, not the emotions. Love involves obedience to God, His plan for us, and an obedience to the permanency of the union. A couple who is living a holy marriage sets their gaze upon God as they strive to follow His directives.

If the couple is not getting closer to God, they are at risk of not only remaining stagnant, but slipping away from God. An extreme result could involve struggling with lust, materialism or treating each other as objects, neglecting each other and taking each other for granted.

What does this discussion of love and marriage have to do with birth? Well, if we acknowledge that marriage is a union that is total and exclusive, we can extend that thinking to the act of childbirth. How so? A baby is the concrete manifestation of a couple's love. Childbirth is the culmination of sex, involving private parts, which infers exclusivity, complete trust, and uninhibition. Women who embrace natural childbirth often prefer to be naked during the final moments of labor. Therefore, birth in its most natural context warrants privacy and exclusivity between partners.

Does this mean that we should not invite third parties to our birth? Childbirth author Marilyn A. Moran would say that midwives, children and others should not be present at birth, which is a private event meant to be shared by husband and wife, exclusively. My preference is sharing the birth experience with my husband and I would reach out to others if we felt a true need or deep desire to include others. I cannot give a prescription for other couples. It's a personal decision that evolves from a philosophy of birth, which is different for each person.

During birth, we are able to give the gift of ourselves to our partner as we trust our partner and experience one of the most intimate moments of our marriage. The childbirth industry has successfully shoved from consciousness any notion that birth is an intimate, private moment. Instead, childbirth is thought of as something to be feared and not revered, something that requires experts and machinery.

During the conjugal act, man and woman rediscover the mystery of Creation. Birthing a child in an intimate way, or unassisted, is also an opportunity to rediscover the mystery of Creation. I can tell you that my first four doctor-delivered hospital births did not allow for the level of spiritual and physical intimacy and awe during childbirth as did my two unassisted births. Gratitude for marriage and family as well as spiritual maturity of men and women in our culture would be greatly enhanced if more people experienced unassisted homebirth.

As I mentioned in the last chapter, it is worth repeating that as birth progresses naturally, couples can relax when there are no delivery room distractions or strangers directing the process. Because there is total privacy between lovers during an intimate birth, it is likely that there will be an exceptional interaction at the birth. Having a child is the most creative thing a couple can do and a baby is a permanent example of the joining of the couple's hearts and minds. If the parents share in the process of making and raising a child, they should have a meaningful sharing at the birth event.

Odds are against a couple trying to achieve a profound union where there are others present at the birth or if the setting is uncomfortable. Intimate birth can be emotionally appealing to the extent that women may lose sight of the physical pain that often accompanies childbirth. No separations between the couple, no small talk or interference from strangers, no hospital employees making requests - what a way to have a baby!

While the couple is strengthening their bond during the birth, they are also beginning parenthood with confidence. By seeing each other in a new situation, and one that requires courage, a special, mutual respect develops. If couples triumph after a birth experience, they can do anything; they are ready to take on the world. Politicians, community and business leaders generally agree that the key to a strong society is strong families. What better place to enhance marital harmony and family unity than with an unassisted homebirth?

I know I might be repetitious, but I want to emphasize the following point because I have experienced it and many others have too: Doctor-delivered hospital birth interferes with the sacredness of the exclusive union between husband and wife. To what extent will depend on at least three factors: whether or not the expectant mother has excessive admiration for the doctor; the level of medical intervention at a birth that could have been eliminated; and the father's level of participation during the birth.

I realize this creates a dilemma for the woman who has confidence, but feels comfortable hiring a doctor and birthing her baby in a hospital. There is no one right or wrong way to have a baby. I will tell you that very few women who have an unassisted homebirth go on to birth a subsequent child in the hospital. On the other hand, it is common for a woman to birth a baby in a hospital or with a midwife at home and to then choose unassisted birth for her next children.

My challenge to you is to thoroughly consider your options, pray about it and make peace with your decisions.

Modern Catholic doctors can be applauded for upholding the dignity of women if they do not prescribe artificial birth control or perform sterilizations or abortions, but they risk interfering in the couple's relationship if they deliver a baby who could have been born without their help.

If we view love as a mutual self-donation between husband and wife, if we believe that human life from the beginning requires a creative, purposeful action by God, and if we believe that unassisted homebirth is an act of love, then unassisted homebirth is a prime example of self-donation and agape love. Marilyn A. Moran believed that birth was a conjugal act in which the husband donates his gift to the wife and nine months later, she presents the gift of the baby. We could say that a doctor-delivered baby is a form of "birth contraception" because it is an artificial way of birthing, and is contrary to how nature intended.

Again, my conclusions are challenging and might seem narrow and opinionated. All I ask is for you to contemplate my perspective.

Any couple who has received the Sacrament of Matrimony might remember the phrase, "Let no man divide what God has joined together." During childbirth, couples are unknowingly divided in the delivery room. The obstetrician takes center stage as the husband sits on the sideline. On the other hand, fathers who travel through forty weeks of pregnancy knowing that they will be the first to touch and see their babies begin family life with a deep emotional attachment and commitment.

In "Theology of the Body," John Paul II says:

"Man and woman express themselves in the measure of the whole truth of the human person the conjugal act signifies not only love, but also potential fecundity. Therefore it cannot be deprived of its full and adequate significance by artificial means. In the conjugal act it is not licit to separate the unitive aspect from the procreative aspect, because both one and the other pertain to the intimate truth of the conjugal act. The one is activated together with the other and in a certain sense the one by means of the other...Therefore, in such a case the conjugal act, deprived of its interior truth because it is artificially deprived of its procreative capacity, ceases also to be an act of love."

John Paul II was talking about marriage and sex here, but I think it is not a far stretch to apply this thinking to childbirth as a sacred and holy act between married couples. We know that a baby is the product of the conjugal act, but let's imagine that birth is a conjugal act. Doctor-delivered birth does not allow for the unitive coming together of husband and wife. Of course the doctor is not going to interfere with the indissolubility of the union, but he is an outsider in the couple's intimate life and should not be part of the couples' birth experience unless there is some medical reason for him to be there.

If we turn to a doctor when we are fraught with worry or fear, we are looking for worldly solutions to alleviate our concerns, solutions that are artificial and solutions that interfere with our interior truth and opportunity to form a deep union with God.

If we look to Jesus for guidance we know that He chose to be born in the most humble and simple of circumstances.

Obstetricians are quick to point out that it was a primitive stable – unsafe and dirty, devoid of modern technology. But Jesus chose the exact time and location. Was He wrong or flawed?

By hiring an obstetrician, we are making compromises in our marital union and with our relationship with God. How? Why? Because we are placing a wedge (a sometimes needed wedge when expectant mothers have major medical concerns) between our trust in God and potential for spiritual growth. A pregnant woman should do everything she can to invite her husband to share the birth as intimately as possible. Allow him to display his strength and valor by serving as a protector and supporter. Fathers are doubly blessed if they are the first to touch, catch or receive their baby. We need to trust in God and summon all the courage we can during childbirth so that we can grow in faith and love.

A holy birth is one in which we are truly united to God and our lovers. Life doesn't get much better than that!

PART III: HOW TO TAKE BACK YOUR BIRTH

CHAPTER 9: YOUR BIRTH WILL BE HOW YOU IMAGINE IT

Pretty powerful statement. I'm suggesting that, to a large extent, your birth is already predetermined by what you think. Your fears, assumptions and visions of your birth have a good chance of being played out in the delivery room or at home.

I've known many women during their pregnancies who I could almost guarantee would be having a C-section, not based on any medical evaluation on my part, but by their attitude, the amount of responsibility they were willing to take for their births, their body image, need for control, and the way they talk about perceived pain.

Albert Einstein once stated that man's greatest gift and power was his imagination. Norman Vincent Peale captured the attention of millions with his "power of positive thinking" theories. His research revealed that those who practiced visualization and affirmation came to believe and therefore actualize what they imagined. It's no surprise that some of the most successful athletes are those whose visualizations have manifested.

While goal setting is important for a satisfying birth experience, dreams during pregnancy can reveal unconscious thoughts and concerns. Dreams are a component of our imaginations manifested in a different manner.

All too often, the body, rather than the mind, is seen as the temple of childbirth. Obstetricians are skilled in the treatment of the body, so it is up to you to fine-tune your spirit and mind. "What the mind can conceive and believe, it can achieve," said the late author and speaker Earl Nightingale.

As we progress through life's journey, most of us gain strength and wisdom. Expectant couples have up to forty weeks to gain trust and courage and to decrease fear and doubt. Some couples use this time more wisely than others. There is a direct relationship between expectations and reality. Expect a thirty-hour labor and you may get a thirty-hour labor! Expect severe pain and your brain will send messages to the rest of your body, which may cause it to freeze up and shut down, increasing the "need" for pain medication.

Aidan Macfarlane, author of "The Psychology of Childbirth" states:

"There seems to be a relation between anxiety, overt or covert, and the length of labor. Uterine dysfunction may also be associated with concealed anxiety. Harry Bakow found that mothers who were anxious during pregnancy and who expressed more concern over the course of their pregnancy more often had babies who got into distress at delivery. Recent studies suggest that women likely to have complications during childbirth are those who during pregnancy, showed concern for the condition of the child, saw their employment as being disrupted, listed a greater number of contact with women who had complicated pregnancies, and described their own mother's health as poor."

Childbirth author Carl Jones has a few resources that can help women enter their birth experiences with tremendous mental strength. He gives specific visualization exercises, describes how to relax, and how to create the optimal birthing environment, whether you choose hospital delivery or homebirth.

In "Unassisted Homebirth: An Act of Love," I show readers the many success stories of men and women who birth with mental strength and courage – how they prepare and the secrets that have helped them achieve successful and peaceful births. Less pain and shorter labors are often the result of powerful imaginations. Goal setting and a positive mental outlook are tools that we all have readily available and they don't cost anything. Accessing your imagination can bring you great rewards. All you need is a little time and effort.

"Engage the imagination, then take it where you will. Where the mind has repeatedly journeyed, the body will surely follow. People go to places they have already been in their minds." – Roy Williams

CHAPTER 10: A SELF-ACTUALIZED BIRTH

"We are all functioning at a small fraction of our capacity to live fully in its total meaning of loving, caring, creating and adventuring. Consequently, the actualizing of our potential can become the most exciting adventure of our lifetime." - Herbert Otto

For years, psychologist Abraham Maslow's theory of self-actualization crept in to my life, first in college, again in graduate school, and then in my working life. From my earliest memories, I have been in search of fulfilling my potential and concerned with becoming a fully functioning person. I longed to join the ranks of the one or two percent of the population (according to Maslow) who are self-actualized.

I believe that my need for self-actualization was met with the birth of my fifth child in 1996. The birth was a very simple, natural event. The only difference was that my husband and I chose to have our baby at home, with no attendants. Our baby was born in the privacy of our bedroom, the same intimate setting as the conception. We were physically, mentally and spiritually prepared for the birth. Yet many people considered our behavior risky and radical.

Upon discovering my pregnancy, I began a search for other couples who decided to intentionally birth their babies in the privacy of their own homes, without assistance. Of the dozens of couples I encountered, there were striking similarities. Men and women often lost track of time during their birth event and experienced birth as effortless. Men who were anxious at the onset of labor were overtaken by a sense of tranquility during the birth. The women who decided to birth in the absence of trained medical experts were well informed about childbirth.

Although most men were somewhat familiar with the anatomy and physiology of birth, cord clamping and responding to minor problems, their instincts during the birth dominated intellectual preparation. When instincts served as their guide, they did not perceive a cord wrapped around the baby's neck as an emergency. Instead, they simply lifted it over the baby's head and helped their wives complete their mission. There was no panic, no sense of effort. They were driven by their inner nature and impulses.

Maslow asserts that, "In states of peak experience, we experience phenomena in their simplicity, 'oughtness,' beauty, goodness, and completeness. There is a lack of strain, an effortlessness, a spontaneity about the experience that is almost overwhelming. Typically there is a lack of space and time. Intense emotions such as wonder, awe, and reverence are felt. During these intense experiences, individuals transcend their own selfishness. Events and objects are perceived as they truly are and are not distorted to meet the experiencer's needs or wishes."

It is difficult, if not impossible to reach a peak birth experience in the hospital. Women must organize themselves mentally while at the same time, orient themselves to their physical surroundings. It is highly unlikely to reach the necessary level of detachment in a setting where there are unfamiliar smells, an uncomfortable room temperature, strangers making demands, and other discomforts. Birth is a medical procedure when it is surrounded by technology and drugs, performed to the staff's convenience, with rules and regulations.

Laboring women are not usually aware of the possibility of a birth orgasm or that birth can be pleasurable. Those couples who have birthed with less distraction or interference have often reported pleasurable birth experiences. Birthing without obstetricians or midwives means birthing with love.

A self-actualized birth is much more likely during an intimate birth. Technological births and medical professionals who orchestrate birth events leave little room for a laboring woman to experience an empowered, authentic birth. It is possible, but a lot of effort and obstacles might need to be overcome. Lovers who take full responsibility for their births have an opportunity to achieve a greater sense of trust and accomplishment.

CHAPTER 11: GOAL SETTING AND PERSISTENCE: WITHOUT THEM, YOU MAY BE SETTING YOURSELF UP FOR DISAPPOINTMENT

We have everything we need to have a successful childbirth experience: our mind, our attitude, and our diligence. Improving our knowledge as we strive for physical, mental and spiritual health during pregnancy will pay off during birth. In addition to a positive attitude, goal setting and persistence are very important.

Successful births are ones where the couple can look back on the event and feel a sense of triumph and confidence. Expectations and goals were met. A question to ask yourself upon discovery of a pregnancy is, "Will I set my own goals or will I relinquish power to others who will make choices for me?"

If you explore what you want from your childbirth event and then make decisions, you are more likely to feel a sense of mastery over pregnancy and birth, rather than mystery, surprise, and confusion. Without clear goals, you could be swept away in the excitement and your goals may end up not being your own, but those of your doctor or midwife.

And what goals am I talking about? Matters such as where to birth your baby, who you would like at your birth, how much technology or intervention you want (during pregnancy and birth), how you will deal with pain, and how you will react when things are not going as planned or visualized.

Goals emerge from assumptions. Doctors are trained to focus on the body. Emphasis is on avoiding pain (through medication) and producing a physically healthy baby. Human beings are much more than the sum of their body parts.

Some new mothers are unable to pinpoint what was missing from their birth experience, but it was because they neglected to participate fully in their births on a psychological, emotional, spiritual and physical level. These elements are all interdependent and contribute to a profound experience.

Here are just a few contrasting goals between expectant moms and doctors. These were mentioned in Chapter 3, but are worth repeating. I've added a few new thoughts.

(1) OPTIMIST MEETS WITH INDIFFERENCE. When an excited mom seeks obstetrical care, she often meets a doctor who is trained (and therefore looking) for a problem to diagnose or treat. Prenatal appointments concentrate on what is going wrong physically rather than encouraging successful behaviors to ensure an empowering birth. Some large OB/Gyn practices have multiple doctors with hundreds of patients they hardly know.

Over the course of several months, health care workers' approach may replace the patient's optimism. Unbeknownst to the patient, she may adopt the doctor's and hospital's goals. Hospital classes prepare couples for birthing according to their policies and rules, i.e., they tell a woman what her goals are and what they expect of her!

Hospitals are known to present birthing preparation classes which teach women avoidance, and in my case in the late 1980's, meaningless breathing exercises, while the Bradley method teaches empowerment at birth. The "better safe than sorry" approach to obstetrical care did not position me to have a thriving pregnancy or empowering birth experience.

(2) PROTECTOR VERSUS ENCOURAGER. In general, men feel a strong need to protect women during vulnerable moments. Problems arise when the protector (doctor) does not fully understand the needs of who he is protecting. A major assumption is that maternity patients need pain medication. Rather than encourage women to deal with pain by avoiding drugs, medication is thrust upon women in labor. Some medical professionals are motivated to protect their jobs, careers or reputations rather than form an alliance with a patient whose goal is a satisfying birth.

(3) WANT VERSUS NEED. Women want to have a baby while doctors and hospitals need to assist at the birth and perform some type of service. The hospital policies may dictate bureaucratic rules rather than what the patient wants or needs. For example, many hospitals do not allow eating during labor, require that birth be in a certain position, or require that C-sections be performed in certain situations or after a certain amount of time has passed.

(4) MATTER OVER MIND. As mentioned before, birth is treated as a medical event rather than a holistic experience. Neglecting the other elements of birth leaves an emptiness, disappointment or memory of pain so that few couples look forward to going through childbirth another time.

In order to have a liberating birth, set a goal that you will not deny your true experience of the emotional, spiritual and psychological expressions at birth. You will then come to realize that drugs, surgery and other unnatural restrictions will get in your way or impede progress. And most people think that technology is superior to nature!

Women are not encouraged to take responsibility for their births because if they did, they would not need the establishment. Submission to authority is expected and the authority often abuses its power, both intentionally and unintentionally. It is up to couples to take some initiative and direct their birth events. Set goals or you will end up with an experience that is not your own.

CHAPTER 12: FIVE SECRETS FOR AN EASIER BIRTH

1. Arrive at the hospital or go into the delivery room well into labor.
2. Strengthen your perineum for birth.
3. Invite a "doula" (labor coach) to your birth.
4. Be quiet.
5. Visualize the baby's passage into the world rather than focus on your own pain.

(1) ARRIVE AT THE HOSPITAL WELL INTO LABOR. Mothers will tell you that labor often includes hours of pain. While some women feel safer laboring in the hospital, there are more freedoms at home, especially during early labor.

The hospital room can be restrictive. Upon arrival, a woman may be checked for dilation, given an IV and hooked up to an Electronic Fetal Monitor. As time progresses, she may be given Pitocin to speed up her labor and the amniotic sac may be broken. Pitocin is a strong drug that often increases the strength and length of contractions and many women are in such excruciating pain that they request more drugs to ease their pain. Often times the body and mind become confused and do not work perfectly together. Over 35% of women who take pain medication (epidurals) end up with C-sections because of the "failure to progress."

In addition to freedom of movement and not being put on a "time clock," other advantages for staying home include: no intrusive or painful pelvic exams, no pressure to take drugs, the right to eat or drink something other than ice chips, and privacy.

(2) One way to decrease the likelihood of a vaginal tear or episiotomy (intentional cut to enlarge the vaginal opening) is to STRENGTHEN THE PERINEUM. In addition to "Kegel" exercises during pregnancy, squatting and tailor-sitting exercises will help strengthen muscles used during birth. Perineal massage is very important and can be practiced during the last six to eight weeks of pregnancy. Although doctors do not educate patients on this technique, information is readily available on how to perform perineal massage.

During birth, your partner or attendant should apply warm compresses to the perineum. A mother who is able to give birth with gravity as her ally (i.e., delivery in a squatting or standing position) will have a 10% less chance of tearing. Do not hurry the birth or be overly aggressive about pushing. Patience is important.

(3) TAKE A CLASS AND /OR HIRE A DOULA. Taking a Bradley childbirth class has helped many couples achieve a natural birth, and a labor support coach (or doula) can contribute to an easier birth. The Journal of American Medical Association has admitted that labor support significantly reduces the incidence of medical interventions, including epidural anesthesia, forceps deliveries and C-sections. Couples who hire coaches tend to have less neonatal complications and a quicker labor.

(4) SILENCE is a very important part of giving birth. Small talk and medical talk often interfere with women's ability to concentrate while in the hospital. Women who want to use their full power at birth need to concentrate and focus. Couples can get the quiet they need simply by asking. Ask that medical staff visits be kept to a minimum, that the door be closed, and that talking be kept to a minimum. Birth is a miracle that transcends reality and couples need quiet time to contemplate the awesome act they are undergoing, the monumental life-changing event taking place, and the intensive task at hand for the next eighteen years.

Silence immediately after birth is respectful to the baby and allows the body, brain and soul to replenish and recover from an altered state of consciousness. Couples are severely shortchanged if they feel they have to perform in the delivery room and maintain some sort of social etiquette because they are in a public place for their private event.

(5) Because the pain is often intense during massive contractions, it is hard for women to get their minds off the pain they are experiencing. In addition to playing some mind games to ease your pain, CONSIDER WHAT THE BABY IS FEELING. Pretend you are the baby making your way into the world. Consider the five senses: How would your body feel? What does it sound like? What do you see? How about taste and smell? How can your mother (you) help you to make this a pleasant experience?

These are just a few secrets for achieving a more pleasurable birth. For dozens more, please refer to "Unassisted Homebirth: An Act of Love" regardless of where you choose to give birth.

CHAPTER 13: THE KEY TO A SUCCESSFUL BIRTH: F.O.C.U.S.

The key to successful birthing can be found in one 5-letter word: FOCUS. Like an Olympic skier who sees every detail of his performance before it occurs, mothers-to-be must have their minds geared toward a successful birth: a birth in which they are in charge; a birth in which they have made decisions (such as the commitment to forego medication or to birth spontaneously in a position that will suit them at the moment); and a birth where they have a determination that goes beyond "wishing," "hoping," or "intending."

The key that will unlock the door to success is found in the word FOCUS: Fortitude, Other People's Opinions, Confidence, Unwavering Determination and Solitude & Surrender.

FORTITUDE is the strength of mind that enables a person to meet danger or bear pain or adversity with courage. We know that minor or major things can go wrong at birth. Most of us assume that intense pain accompanies birth. The key is to have the courage to know that in most cases, more than 95% of the time, things occur normally and without a hitch. It's up to you to decide whether or not you will focus on the positive or obsess, fear and worry about the remote possibilities.

OTHER PEOPLE'S OPINIONS. Childbirth classes aren't enough. A written birth plan isn't enough. In order to strengthen this focus, women need to reach deep down and feel the energy begin to flow. Talk with women who have had great, empowering births. If you can't find anyone in your local area who has experienced an extraordinary birth, make the internet your friend.

Whatever you read or watch regarding birth should be positive and life-affirming. Detach and disregard the birth horror stories. They coax you back to fear, helplessness and hopelessness. They will only serve to redirect your focus to thinking that conventional childbirth is appealing and doctor-managed birth is necessary. Your goal is a woman-centered birth, baby-centered birth, and/or couple-centered birth, not an institutional directed birth. You deserve more and are meant to have the most dignified birth possible. Carefully choose the person(s) you want at your birth.

Do not disregard the inner work you may need to do if you are strongly influenced by other women in your life: your mother, close female friends and relatives. Their opinions might infiltrate your mind in ways that can affect the upcoming birth of your baby.

The focus should be on your internal power, not the external system. The system is there to aid you should you need it, but not do it for you. Don't be tempted to relinquish power to others.

CONFIDENCE. Concern yourself with increasing your confidence in yourself and your body's ability to birth your baby. Prayer can be the answer to insecurity and doubt. Continue your research and childbirth reading. As time progresses, think of yourself as gaining valuable ammunition as you form a protective shield from negative outside influences. Learn to discern which outside influences can be helpful.

Visualize being assertive in the delivery room (if you choose to give birth in a hospital) or with your midwife. How will you cast away those unwelcome voices of discouragement during the final moments of birth? Confidence comes from believing and knowing that you'll do fine and that millions of women have given birth before you. You are not alone.

The mind is what often holds us back. Ask any athlete. Many times they will tell you that the body is able, but the mind can sabotage performance. Consider the idea that you are only as safe as you think. You're only as safe as you personally prepare yourself. Some physical circumstances may be beyond your control, but you have enormous mental power; tap into it.

UNWAVERING DETERMINATION. Set goals, know what you want and what you definitely don't want. You must commit yourself. For example, if you don't intend to have an epidural, develop other coping strategies for pain management. All the education and planning in the world is useless if you don't have unwavering determination and a commitment to follow-through. This quality will set you apart from the rest. Unwavering determination is 100% mental preparation before you get to your fortieth week of pregnancy.

SOLITUDE & SURRENDER. If you haven't spent much time in solitude, the last few weeks of your pregnancy are definitely the time to do so. In fact, you would be wise to find more time for solitude and pleasurable activities at the beginning of your third trimester. Try to spend little or no time with negative people. Avoid activities that cause you stress or make you uneasy. Don't make excuses that you are too busy to shift the focus of your daily routine to your pregnancy and upcoming birth. You have almost complete freedom in where you want to direct your thoughts and actions. Successful childbirth requires concentration. Practicing solitude will make you stronger and enable you to surrender during the important task of giving birth.

CONCLUSION. I'm not making an outrageous statement when I admit that I LIVE to swim. Several times a week, you'll find me in the pool swimming laps, focusing and visualizing all of the good things that I plan on doing or that I "know" will happen. I'm at one with my thoughts and body. There is an inner peace that no one can take away, a smoothness and joy in life. No worries or fears, just calmness and creative thoughts.

You need to find this inner peace. When you focus, there's no stopping you. You are birthing from within and no one can take you off your path. Nothing will deter you from your goals and dreams.

All of the steps of FOCUS are intended to give you an inner conviction. Some women do not consider or care about what it takes to have a successful birth. Their focus is on safety and putting the birth behind them. I would venture to guess that your outcome will be very close to what you focus on. I invite you to take this key which will unlock the door to your success. What are you waiting for?

PART IV: AUTONOMOUS BIRTH

CHAPTER 14: WHAT'S THE BIG DEAL ABOUT NATURAL CHILDBIRTH?

What is Natural Childbirth? Natural childbirth means different things to different people. Some women consider a vaginal birth a natural birth. Others say a natural birth is one which did not include any drugs whatsoever. However, a baby is not born completely natural if the mother is restrained by a fetal monitor, told what position to deliver the baby, when to push, or limited by what she can eat or drink.

A completely natural birth would be one in which the baby arrived on nature's time table, without the aid of medical instruments, machines or medication. In addition, the couple would choose who they wanted at their birth and what position in which to give birth. This is almost non-existent in a hospital setting. Statistics indicate that less than 1% of American couples choose homebirths, and less than 5% choose settings (such as a birth center) where professionals offer encouragement for non-medicated deliveries.

I cannot discuss the benefits of natural childbirth without presenting the potential harmful effects of medication.

Because drugs often dull physical and mental pain, a woman is not at full strength during delivery or in full control of her mental and physical capacities. Natural childbirth requires confidence, responsibility, faith and trust in nature, and education of the birth process.

Many obstetric patients want to be relieved of pain and suffering and are less concerned with the short-term harm and potential long-term effects of drugs or surgery, while natural childbirth patients rely on personal strength and power. They train themselves how to cope with temporary discomfort and are more likely to end up with shorter labors, less blood loss and a smoother convalescence. Natural childbirth also leads to closer attachment and longer breastfeeding.

Because babies are born healthier and there are no injuries or death as a result of medication complications, natural childbirth is the safest way to birth a baby. Nursery room nurses will tell you that there is a noticeable difference in the alertness, breathing and behavior of newborns who were not subjected to an epidural or C-section.

As drugs numb the pain, women miss an opportunity for a physical peak experience that is often described by natural childbirth patients. Some authors have stated that a birth climax is essential and that a mother who has missed it and had a passive, frigid birth because of anesthetics or local injections is emotionally in a state of expectancy. She looks at her child and experiences no euphoria, no sense of exhilaration.

One might think more women would desire natural childbirth. Well, guess what? Fear and conformity (emotional feelings) often override common sense (logical reasoning). It is easier to blend into society and adopt conforming behaviors than to seek a truly satisfying experience. Institutional pressure or procedures leave many women with an unpleasant delivery who could have birthed naturally.

Some Americans turn to drugs to escape the pains of life. Illegal narcotics, alcohol, Ritalin, Prozac, antidepressant drugs, or other drugs may offer temporary relief, but bring with them side effects and consequences. Opioid addiction and other pain medication addiction has reached epidemic levels.

How you deal with pain, your beliefs about birth, and level of fear will affect your choices. I suspect that the unborn would unanimously choose natural childbirth, but many women do not feel comfortable with an unmedicated birth.

Women can have a hard time surrendering to a completely natural or raw birth because they prefer a life of order and control. While neatness, planning and maintaining order are valued, flexibility and spontaneity are equally significant. Girls are taught that maintaining appearance and control are revered, so you can see that an uninhibited birth is contrary to years of indoctrination.

In addition to avoiding pain, an unspoken reason women accept epidurals is that they don't want to display uninhibited or primitive behavior. After all, their legs are spread exposing their private parts in a room full of strangers. They don't want to be seen groaning, moaning, and sweating. When we can completely trust, when we can surrender and not be afraid of being vulnerable - those are the moments of greatest satisfaction and pleasure. And those are the times where wisdom, enlightenment and faith often come pouring into our lives. Life is about taking risks and facing it with courage.

Choosing natural birth is an act of courage. We are put on Earth so that we can contribute to our world and in order to do that, we need to grow in love, courage and wisdom. One way to gain courage is to face challenges. Giving birth not only perpetuates the human race, but gives women an opportunity to become more courageous, an important quality for successful parenting. Welcoming a raw birth reveals strength, strength that is crucial for a meaningful life.

CHAPTER 15: "JUST IN CASE"

As an unassisted homebirth advocate, I am often asked, "Why wouldn't you want someone at your birth...just in case?"

That question presumes that childbirth is risky and dangerous and that a skilled expert should be present. Childbirth was designed to be a natural process, and most mothers and babies emerge alive and healthy. However, a majority of women have allowed the natural progression of childbirth to be aided, and sometimes thwarted by drugs and surgery. There's no reason why more couples who are mentally and physically prepared could not birth their baby at home.

At some point in history, women and men became convinced that birth was dangerous and required experts. Women are not encouraged to have complete confidence in their bodies, nor do they fully trust their intuition. We relinquish our inner power to some "expert" who brings with him or her past experiences, medical training, and monetary goals.

Women are taught to fear birth, to fear pain, and to assume that something will go wrong. We are taught to conform to the medical manner of giving birth, disregarding that birth is a sexual experience.

What is a hospital or doctor going to do for you? Life-saving equipment is only needed in a small percentage of cases. Yet, many pregnant couples assume they may need that equipment. Birthing in a high-tech environment tempts the professionals to use that equipment. Early birth researchers from the 1980's, including Dr. David Stewart, Dr. Lewis Mehl, Sheila Kitzinger, and Robbie Davis-Floyd knew long ago that technology was and is not always employed properly. It may be overused or misused.

What will a skilled midwife do for you while birthing at home? She will bring years of experience and expertise dealing with dozens or hundreds of births. Perhaps she will check dilation or use an instrument to monitor the baby's heart rate. She may bring a calm, reassuring demeanor to a birth where parents are somewhat trepid. But a true medical emergency might require hospitalization. Couples can learn what to do in the cases of a cord wrapped tightly around the baby's neck, hemorrhage, or shoulder dystocia. A couple can learn CPR or rent an oxygen tank and learn how to treat a baby who is not breathing. And if a couple live close enough to the hospital, they can call 911 or go to the hospital.

If you live your life with optimism that you will fall into the 95% category for a truly safe, uneventful birth, then you will be comfortable birthing without relying on technology. If your thoughts and energy are channeled toward the small percentage who truly need medical assistance, then you should either work on alleviating fear and addressing your concerns, or birth in the hospital and be grateful for the expertise.

Proper prenatal care may identify the need for a hospital delivery. Following one's intuition may reveal that the most comfortable place for birth is in the hospital. A woman I know was planning an unassisted birth and was experiencing close, consistent, contractions for five days. Realizing that there was no medical emergency, but frustrated because she wasn't progressing, she decided to go to the hospital. Within a few hours, her amniotic sac broke and the baby was born. Her place of comfort was in the hospital.

Why go to all the trouble of taking the risk of birthing on your own? First of all, childbirth is not a high risk when a couple is physically and mentally healthy. But more importantly, BIRTH, LIKE CONCEPTION, IS A LOVER'S INTERLUDE REQUIRING PRIVACY FOR AN AUTHENTIC EXPRESSION OF SEXUALITY. If we take the medical emphasis out of birth and replace it with the idea that birth is sexual and sensual, we see that there is little room for third parties.

I know I am proposing an unusual idea, but just think about a world where more couples trusted the process of pregnancy and birth and gave birth freely. Husbands would have the opportunity to receive (or catch) their babies, which enhances emotional maturity and reverence for sexuality. And women would actually enjoy childbirth.

Many couples who choose to birth at home are uneasy about all of the medical interventions and complications that occur in the hospital because of a "just in case" attitude. Hospital classes teach parents to prepare for a C-section JUST IN CASE the doctor determines it is necessary. Did you know that birth researchers say that the true need for C-sections is 5%, yet our national average is over 33%? Most women are convinced that their C-section was a true necessity. "In MY case, I needed to have a C-section. If we attempted a homebirth, someone would have died."

First of all, it is only an assumption that death would have occurred. Also, the labor scenario in the hospital is quite different from labor and birth at home. A baby who is "stuck" after two hours of pushing in the delivery room is almost always inside a mother who is lying on a table. Women at home get into squatting or standing positions.

What often becomes an emergency in the hospital is because of what is done in the hospital. For example, thousands of women are given Pitocin to speed up their labor every day in hospitals around the world. Contractions

111

intensify, prompting the request for an epidural. Epidurals commonly interfere with the mother's ability to push and work in synchronization with the childbirth process. Then labor stalls.

The fetal monitors indicate a heart rate problem or baby in distress and after two hours of pushing, the doctor will determine that the mom's pelvis is too small for the baby to pass. A C-section is performed and couple is grateful for the life-saving C-section! Many C-sections do not constitute a successful birth, but a failed vaginal delivery. The system fails when 33% of births end in C-sections rather than the 5% true need.

We should all consider the "just in case" or "what if" scenarios in our lives, but we would be better off if we took a fearless, objective approach and kept our sights on the probability that things will go well rather than worry about the possible tragedies in life. And, if you're planning a hospital birth, have you ever asked, "What if I don't make it on time?" "What if the baby is born in the car?" "What if severe weather prevents me from making it to the hospital?" "Am I ready to give birth at home, just in case?"

CHAPTER 16: THE CASE FOR UNASSISTED HOMEBIRTH

Childbirth can be one of the greatest joys on earth. The birth of a baby marks the beginning of parenthood and is central to womanhood, personhood, couplehood.

Bearing a child makes a strong impact on a woman's sense of femininity. Her birth experience will remain with her for a lifetime. Memory of her birth event can be summoned to conscious thought within seconds. Few other experiences in life can be remembered so easily and vividly.

One of the problems with our culture is that we do not like the act of birth. We avoid it. We fear it. We endure it. The secret to a satisfying birth is to embrace it, not escape from it. If we prepare physically, mentally, and spiritually and then welcome birth as a beautiful event, childbirth becomes a whole new opportunity for joy. Unassisted homebirth presents an opportunity to experience a pleasurable birth.

A father is profoundly influenced by childbirth. Birth is especially meaningful when he accepts responsibility for an event which has been in everyone's domain but his for over a century. A father experiences great joy when he is the first to see, touch and hold his own child. He will instantly know that no doctor, midwife or other person should be the one to accept this new miracle in their hands.

Our decisions and actions about birth are based on cultural methods. We submit to established procedures, often neglecting to question convention. Those who question convention and are unhappy with the status quo are often led to alternative methods.

On August 3, 1996, I gave birth to our fifth child, Millicent. It was a very simple, natural event. The only difference was that we chose to have our baby at home, with no attendants. Our baby was born in the privacy of our bedroom, the same intimate setting as the conception. We were prepared for the birth, yet many people considered our behavior risky and radical. Thousands of other couples across the country have discovered that unassisted homebirth offers many advantages compared to institutional birth.

SAFETY. When I was preparing for my homebirth, researchers such as Sheila Kitzinger, Lewis Mehl, David Stewart and Carol Balizet cited evidence that reveal planned homebirth as significantly safer than hospital birth. Today, evidence and statistics can confuse expectant parents. The biases in the studies are still prevalent. However, today as well as decades ago, a much larger percentage of babies die in the hospital than at home.

DRUGS. The implementation of technology and drugs are often imposed on women who desire a natural birth. Tests and equipment do not always serve the best interests of every birthing woman. Most hospital births include some type of drug, whether it is Pitocin, epidural or anesthesia. Drugs carry risks and are harmful to the unborn and newly born even though women are told that the current drugs are better and safer than ever before. Many women are coaxed into receiving drugs rather than persuaded to avoid them. Childbirth is big business and money is often a motivator to perform more tests and surgeries. Profits are often sought at the expense of providing an environment for a satisfying birth. Drug use is also prevalent in a culture that seeks to escape and avoid pain and discomfort.

Drugs should be avoided during normal vaginal births because they interfere with the brain-body chemistry before, during and after birth; they affect immediate breastfeeding success; they affect the alertness and energy level of the mother and baby; and they effect postpartum attachment and bonding. Those who choose to birth at home do not resort to drugs, but often incorporate visualization, prayer, perineal massage or herbs and homeopathic remedies.

CONTROL. You can be in control of your birth at home. There are no time limits, birthing positions or required hospital policies. Couples are free to eat, move, sing or make love within the privacy of their own home.

SELF-CONFIDENCE. An unassisted birth requires that partners rely upon themselves rather than an expert. When we depend on ourselves and take responsibility, we grow in faith and confidence. Self-sufficiency during birth results in an alert and empowered state of mind, qualities necessary for a successful, productive life.

RITE OF PASSAGE. The birth of a child is perhaps the most significant event in a couple's life together. People who are fully involved in their child's birth often achieve a high level of satisfaction, sense of balance and completion. New mothers and fathers can begin their parenting journey with confidence and pride.

DECIDING IF UNASSISTED HOMEBIRTH IS RIGHT FOR YOU

I cannot determine whether or not someone should have an unassisted homebirth, nor am I an expert on birth. I only know what seems right and appropriate for me. Couples are encouraged to do their own assessment based on the current pregnancy and by considering previous pregnancies and births. A safe, healthy delivery should be the goal of all pregnancies. A birth event should not be an attention getting event or rebellious statement, or worse, a situation which would put the mother's or baby's life in jeopardy.

Unassisted homebirth works well for the woman who is physically and mentally strong, has a basic knowledge of labor and birth, and embraces natural childbirth. We are not trying to act as our own obstetricians or mimic what goes on during high tech hospital births.

In addition to external factors, there is little room for fear or ignorance when attempting an unassisted homebirth. Intuitive "gut" feelings may be telling you one thing, while your logic and reasoning may be steering you in another direction. Severe problems throughout pregnancy may signal that you need a physician's care. This is not a failure on your part, but simply an indication that you may need an experienced caregiver.

Ask "why." Upon discovery of a pregnancy, couples can determine what they want from their birth experience and ask why they need to submit to a series of tests, appointments and rules. One of the worst things a pregnant woman can do is to arrive at an obstetrician's office with no goal in mind. Couples are in a better position to enjoy their birth experiences when they set goals, take responsibility and thoroughly think through their options.

The reason couples are disappointed with their births stems from our cultural approach to birth. Few people question why we choose OB/Gyns and hospitals, preferring instead to conform to conditions where they must leave the nest to add to it, give birth in a painful position while hooked up to equipment, and push a baby out into the world in front of strangers. It never occurs to some people that birth could be a private event and that it can be sexy and pleasurable.

PREPARING FOR UNASSISTED HOMEBIRTH

Each couple will have unique problems and fears to face. Some of the issues that arise include: What do we do about prenatal and postpartum care? What supplies should we have ready? What do we do in an emergency? When do we cut the cord? What do we do with the placenta? What if the baby dies? How do you deal with close friends and relatives who oppose your birth plans?

Answers to these questions come as couples talk to others who have had unassisted homebirths and as they research natural childbirth. I was almost halfway through my pregnancy before I found information on unassisted homebirth and others in my area who actually had unassisted homebirths. Some people may prefer to seek information on the internet rather than search for local residents who are supportive of unassisted homebirth.

There are several resources that can help you prepare for a homebirth - more today than when I was planning my first unassisted birth in 1996. Blogs and videos are plentiful. There are a handful of books and an abundance of personal stories lovingly shared on the internet.

When I was preparing for birth, I came across many excellent resources on homebirth. In 1996, three books that were most helpful to me included: Sheila Kitzinger's "Homebirth: The Essential Guide to Giving Birth Outside of the Hospital," Marilyn A. Moran's, "Birth and the Dialogue of Love," and Gregory White's "Emergency Childbirth: A Manual." Soon after I gave birth, I came across Laura Kaplan Shanley's "Unassisted Childbirth," an excellent and inspiring resource. Today, support on the internet for unassisted homebirth makes it easy to connect with like-minded people.

You conceived your child out of love; why not bear your child the same way? If we let birth happen in the privacy of our own homes, there would be an increase of marital closeness, personal confidence, mother and baby bonding, and family attachment. Politicians, community and business leaders generally agree that the key to a strong society is strong families. What better place to start with marital harmony and family unity than with an unassisted homebirth?

CHAPTER 17: THE POWER OF SILENCE

Blood, sweat, tears of joy and pain, saliva, mucous, vomit, urine, bowel movements. Almost every bodily release occurs during labor, resulting in the final adrenaline-packed moment of the birth release. Add to this scenario the emotions of love, anticipation, anxiety and stress and you have a physically and emotionally intense event that can be best understood and appreciated only in silence.

As a woman nears stage two of labor, the pushing phase, she is usually experiencing pain or at least massive pressure of the baby moving out into the world. In many instances, she does not want to be bothered with a lot of noise, conversation or demands. The same is true in those few magical minutes right after the birth. Yet most deliveries occur in brightly lighted rooms, filled with people scurrying about their business, making mundane conversation. The baby is treated as an object to be examined rather than a person to be immediately loved.

Silence allows the body, brain and soul to replenish itself as it tries to recover from an altered state of consciousness. Silence, which is much easier to capture at home than in the hospital, allows fathers to contemplate their contribution and importance during birth and as a parent. Home allows you to transcend reality, while unfamiliar and anxiety-provoking people and places invade your silent space. Recovery time following the birth event varies for each person. Five minutes, twenty minutes, or a few hours of quiet time is critical for making the transition from pregnancy to parenthood, from a couple to a family. Any distractions or separations during this sensitive period can affect the early days as a new family unit, and jeopardize the chance for a successful rite of passage.

Experts have agreed that if left to nature, many births would occur in the early morning hours, when most people are asleep. This quiet time of the day is nature's way of providing silence for birth. Many babies are conveniently born during normal business hours. Some women make appointments for inductions or C-sections. Aidan Macfarlane, author of "The Psychology of Childbirth," points to a study of 601,222 spontaneous deliveries. He noticed that there was a peak between 3:00 and 4:00 A.M., the time when a woman is likely to be in a peaceful emotional state, in quiet, comfortable surroundings. The onset of labor often begins during this time period.

Birth requires patience and trust. Patience and trust enter the lives of those who are open to it. Laboring women need time and space for concentration, which is best done in the absence of noise.

It was very liberating for me to give birth at home with only my husband. I have always known the importance of silence, and finally figured out how to ensure silence at the birth of my baby. At home I did not have to exert effort to achieve silence, but entering an altered state of consciousness during my hospital births required a lot of mental work. The only silence I had was based on my ability to retreat within myself.

Whether we give birth in the hospital or at home, we must actively pursue silence so that we can concentrate as well as recover from the intensity of birth. If we can clear our minds and incorporate more silence into daily living, perhaps we can approach our lives with more meaning and intensity.

CHAPTER 18: TOP TEN REASONS TO BIRTH AT HOME

1. You don't have to leave the nest to add to it.
2. You have control over your labor and birth.
3. The father is intimately involved rather than a passive observer on the sidelines.
4. Your birth will be surrounded by love as opposed to strangers and equipment.
5. No one ridicules you, hurries you or coaxes you to take drugs.
6. You are more apt to have a safer birth.
7. You are more likely to experience a pleasurable birth.
8. No one will treat the baby as an object (poking, weighing, measuring, taken away for testing and experimentation).
9. You are likely to have less postpartum depression.
10. You will experience tremendous awe and reverence for life. There is a greater likelihood of achieving a high level of fulfillment.

CHAPTER 19: WHY A "RAW BIRTH" IS HARD TO ACHIEVE

Many women have a hard time surrendering to a completely natural or raw birth because they prefer a life of order and control. It's natural and desirable for us to want our environments to be safe, clean and orderly. We feel a sense of mastery if we have a certain amount of control and freedom. Disruptions to this control are barely tolerable.

While neatness, planning and maintaining order are important, flexibility and spontaneity are equally important. Because girls are taught that maintaining appearance and control are primary values, an uninhibited birth is contrary to years of socialization.

Avoiding a raw birth could be considered avoidance. We are put on Earth so that we can contribute to our world as we prepare for our next life, and in order to do that, we need to grow in love, courage and wisdom. One way to gain courage is to face challenges.

The purpose of giving birth not only perpetuates the human race, but gives women an opportunity to become more courageous. It is courageous to go against the mainstream and to overcome fear of giving birth. Welcoming a raw birth reveals strength, strength that is crucial for a meaningful life.

PART V: SUCCESS

CHAPTER 20: SHARING OUR BEAUTIFUL BIRTH STORIES WITH OTHERS

Those of us who have experienced the power and bliss of an unassisted birth are sometimes frustrated when we can't share our birth stories with other women. They are often not able (1) to get beyond their assumptions and fear of birth (2) to avoid comparing your birth with their birth, and / or (3) to get beyond conventional thinking and years of programming that birth is painful and potentially dangerous.

What often ends up happening? We begin to tell them of our glorious, simple, drug-free experience and they say things that seem to halt the momentum of where we'd like to take the conversation, which is to the "meat" of the beauty of our birth experience. Most likely you've heard comments such as, "Wow! You were lucky!…I could never do that…My husband / partner would never do that…How could you give birth without an epidural?…That's not for me…"

Be mindful that many women need to heal from a disappointing birth experience. Your conversation should never be imposing, boastful, or shared with people who might not appreciate it or be ready to hear it. Don't share your story for your benefit; it is a gift for your listener.

First, (1) PARAPHRASE and REFLECT back what they said rather than react by defending or explaining your position. Imagine that you're playing tennis and you are simply returning the ball to their side of the net. Don't allow them to return the ball to you until they explain their original statement or hesitation about unassisted birth.

Examples: A. "So you're saying that you might be interested in a homebirth, but your husband isn't? (Then go on to Step 2 below: PROBE) Why do you think that is?"

"You seem to think that a homebirth is for the most part, luck. PROBE: How so?"

"You could never have a homebirth. PROBE: Why not?"

"Birth without an epidural. PROBE: Why not?"

Step 2: PROBE. Your "opponent" has made a one or two sentence statement that you've paraphrased. Keep the ball on their side of the net until they've backed up or explained their position. They might not expect to have to do this, so give them some time for dialogue and try to draw out what's behind their concern (could it be fear? ignorance? conformity? something else?).

If your friend (tennis opponent) seems to be uncomfortable, uncooperative or ready to end the conversation, you'll have to decide if it's time to wind down the conversation at this point or PROBE further. One example that may be too confrontational, but will give you the information you need: "Something seems to be unsettling about this topic for you. Do you want to talk about it? Would you like to hear my story or are we pretty much through talking about this?" Or, replace sentence two with, "I'd love to share my birth story with you sometime. Just let me know if and when you'd like to hear it."

If she truly cares and is engaged in the conversation, you will be able to continue with Step 3: EDUCATE and ENLIGHTEN. This is not to be confused with "Lecture and Lead." You are gently giving people new ideas to consider.

Don't be too bashful to present startling facts about what can go wrong in the hospital, the dangers of drugs, the violations of medical birth (being hooked up to monitors, confined to the bed, etc.)

Be armed with three or four brief and obvious doctor-caused horror stories to counter their horror stories. Your stories should illustrate the dangers of doctor-managed hospital births. Or better yet, continue probing each particular horror story that they present to you, and focus on what they are communicating. Chances are, they won't be able to back up their one-line fear statements.

Proceed delicately, especially if your friend is talking about her past birth. Education and enlightenment is intended to equip her for the future since she can't go back and correct or relive a disappointing birth. Be careful not to get defensive or arrogant here either. You're simply helping someone come to a new understanding and it's best to be non-threatening and non-confrontational.

Many women will not progress to this step. Maybe they are not ready or not interested. Consider yourself successful if you've made it through Step 2. However, if the dialogue is pleasantly continuing, you might be ready for Step 4: SHARE YOUR BIRTH STORY.

Can you believe it? In the past, you wanted to go directly to this step, but most conventional thinkers aren't ready to hear what you so desperately want to share. Now their hearts and minds may be primed, thanks to you for helping them to progress to this point.

There still might be some hesitation on her part, but I recommend you jump right in, open up and share the excitement. Your enthusiasm is bound to make an impact.

Concluding thoughts: (1) PARAPHRASE (2) PROBE (3) EDUCATE and ENLIGHTEN (4) SHARE YOUR BIRTH STORY. Be open to adverse comments during Step 1; be truly engaged (and not defensive) so your probing can be effective during Step 2. Do not advance to Step 3 unless they seem ready and willing. Present brief and factual statements when you are trying to educate and enlighten others. During Step 4, watch for their feedback to determine how detailed you want to get.

Please write, email or call me and let me know your success, challenges or comments regarding this process or one you are already implementing. It's important for us to share our stories lovingly, with the goal that more women will cherish their birth experiences in the future.

CHAPTER 21: WHAT IS SUCCESS?

What is success? What constitutes success? How do you know if you are successful? Can you describe a successful person?

Everyone will have a different definition. Is success mainly measured by salary? What about fame, talent, material possessions? Who would you say is more successful: Mother Teresa or Bill Gates? Donald Trump or Socrates? Thomas Edison or Hugh Hefner? How about a Hollywood superstar who's had a few marriages and mal-adjusted adult children? OJ Simpson or your blue-collar friend whose three children have respectable low-paying jobs, but have extremely happy marriages and families? Or, are they all successful?

Is success measurable? Are the more successful people those who have a higher salary? How about CEOs of large corporations and professionals who earn more than seven figures a year? Peaceful, charitable people or selfish prosperous braggarts? Maybe we don't need to polarize choices; maybe there is a large spectrum and perhaps success is in the eye of the beholder. Where do values fit? Do personal standards, virtues and character have anything to do with success? Do winners need these qualities?

I believe that the following qualities contribute to success: self-discipline; authenticity and integrity; passion; reason;

common-sense; quick, yet focused decision-making skills; physical and mental endurance to sustain hardship and suffering; stamina to overcome that which is repulsive or frightening; ability to commit for the long term, and at the same time, knowing when to make a change or bold choice; strong communication skills, both verbal and written, among many others.

I have seen and experienced many incidences of "isolated individualism." What I mean is that many people do not seem to place a high value on interdependence with others, which is vital in forming healthy relationships and strong communities. How many people do not even know their immediate neighbors? How many people choose to do things on their own, when there could be a rich exchange of ideas and resources simply by cooperating and coordinating with others?

Taking this to the extreme, we could say that families aren't failing, but modernism is to the extent that there is an emphasis on narcissistic goals. Emphasis on personal gratification can be destructive. What many well-meaning Americans don't realize is that as the father or couple continue their quest for more success in the workplace or more money for the family, they may be neglecting to be fully "present" in their children's lives. Business travel and extra hours at the office or on the job take away time from the marriage and family.

People believe that QUALITY time is more important than QUANTITY time, but relationships form over a period of time, which involves quantity.

The American Heritage Dictionary defines success as the "achievement of something desired, planned or attempted; having a favorable outcome." Let's say you did everything you could to avoid a C-section, but discovered that the baby was in a transverse position. Perhaps you could not find a skilled person to help manipulate the transverse position, precipitating the need for a C-section. Your birth would be successful if you did all you could and believed the outcome was favorable.

What is a successful birth? If your expectations were fulfilled and your deepest desires were met, then we could say you had a satisfying birth. If you are content with your birth experience and feel that it was emotionally and physically gratifying, you're probably satisfied with your birth.

All six of my births were successful, but the two most satisfying include one homebirth and one hospital birth. You can read about the birth of my fifth child in "Unassisted Homebirth: An Act of Love." The birth had all of the elements I've been talking about throughout this book and in the above paragraphs. The birth of my third child, Hilary, was very satisfying, mainly because I arrived at the hospital ten minutes before she was born and experienced very little labor and no pain.

It's not up to me to determine what a satisfying and successful birth means to you. I can give you general guidelines, but in the end, you will make the final determination because your plans, desires and preferences will be different from mine.

Although my preference for childbirth is unassisted birth, your preference will emerge from your philosophy of birth. If you choose a hospital birth, I suggest you assert your intentions during your birth or hire a doula to advocate your desires along with you.

In "Success for Dummies," Zig Ziglar summarizes success: (1) Success begins with the desire to be successful and the conviction that you can be successful. (2) Then, and only then, do you make plans to reach that specific objective of achieving success. (3) After you make plans, you must be willing to commit to them. (4) But no responsible person makes a commitment until he or she has a reasonable plan of action to fulfill that commitment.

Ziglar describes characteristics that contribute to success. They include: conviction, persistence, commitment, discipline, hard work, heredity, integrity, environment, character, humor, luck, consistency, faith, passion, connections and love for what you do.

As you can see, preparation, contemplation, confidence and goal setting figure prominently in a successful birth. With childbirth education classes available on-line and in most communities, it's easy to find the resources you need. It can be difficult being assertive, especially when your values and ideas are very different from others. However, you will not be disappointed if you follow-through on your inner desires. "Nothing ventured, nothing gained" is applicable to childbirth and your success.

CONCLUDING THOUGHTS

I've given you a lot to think about. I'm not asking you to believe my conclusions based on my personal observations and experiences. I am asking that you think about birth in ways you may not have considered – ways that have not been presented to you. Scrutinize and analyze the system before you enter it or get enveloped into it. Do not allow yourself to be swallowed into it if you choose hospital birth. Do your best to make the institution serve you.

While technology is beneficial for those who need it, it often becomes a substitute for human effort, patience and tolerance. Technology employed at birth can also be used to control the event. During birth, it is imperative to surrender to the rhythms of the event as it unfolds. From my experience in talking with hundreds of women who have given birth, those who seem to enjoy their birth experiences are those who have had a more natural birth and those who have had an autonomous birth.

Breastfeeding success and initial mother-infant bonding satisfaction is often reported by those who have had a more natural childbirth experience. Women who develop confidence during pregnancy by listening to their inner voice and yearnings begin parenting with patience and acceptance.

Respond to the environment and task at hand rather than try to exert so much control.

A key to having a satisfying birth is to take control by making decisions based on your inner yearnings, as you go through pregnancy and prepare for birth. You hold the keys to success and happiness. Your decisions and actions are what you have power over and it's up to you to lay the foundation for your birth experience. Notice how I did not say that the outcome is what defines success. There are some factors beyond our control. What we can do is create an environment to foster a desirable outcome and if things do not go as planned, it is important to regroup and adopt a positive attitude and spirit of forgiveness.

Your body houses your spirit and emotions, so be careful about looking outward for inner guidance. Getting in touch with your maternal instinct should be an ongoing process that continues into parenting.

Consider these questions: Is there any one truth about birth? Why do hospital delivery rooms mimic the home? Is this recognition that birth should be private? Would you like more privacy during your birth? Are you willing to make decisions and take actions based on your inner yearnings? Do you have a vision or dream for your birth experience? Do you want complete freedom for your birth or are you more comfortable with a system that helps shape your birth?

If you have desires for your childbirth experience, I suggest that you fully commit to doing all that you can in anticipation of your vision. You will not be sorry. But you may have regrets if you deny your inner voice by falling prey to the cultural hypnosis regarding traditional childbirth.

If you condition your body and mind for success and then believe that you are entitled to the birth of your intentions, you will have a greater likelihood of attaining it. Decide now that you will find coping mechanisms that do not include resorting to an epidural during labor. Decide now that you will take care of yourself to the best of your ability during pregnancy.

So much is possible for you as you prepare for childbirth. The birth of your child is a defining moment in your life and the life of the new baby. It is the beginning of a new generation. Do not conform to others' expectations as you go through such an incredible experience – your experience.

Generate out of your imagination, not your past. Do not let your fears keep you from progressing on a path that your inner voice is nudging you toward. Remember, love can transform fear.

Birth is not only an act of giving, but an act of revelation. Who you are will be revealed during your birth experience. Stand tall and embrace your strength during your birth. You are here to contribute something unique to the human race and one of the greatest challenges that will test a woman's mental and physical strength is the act of childbirth. Take charge of your birth so that it can be everything you've dreamed it would be.

ABOUT THE AUTHOR

Lynn M. Griesemer is a nationally known author and earned the highest award given by Toastmasters International, the Distinguished Toastmasters Medal (DTM), in 2006, after less than five years of membership. She designed "Speaking Made Easy: A Public Speaking Program for Middle School Students" and "Speak Up!: A Public Speaking Program for Young Adults" and served as the primary instructor to hundreds of children.

Lynn homeschooled her six children from 1994-2016 and is a former Human Resources Manager and Army Officer. She received her B.A. in Psychology from Boston University and M.S. in Human Resources Management and Development from Chapman University. She has written books on public speaking, marriage and childbirth.

Lynn is an outspoken critic of traditional American childbirth practices and believes there are many alternatives that women can choose in order to have a better birth experience. She is author of Unassisted Homebirth: An Act of Love (1998) and creator of the CD "Your Body Your Birth: Secrets for a Satisfying and Successful Birth" (2007).

Lynn is focusing her efforts on Marriage Coaching, and writing books on marriage. With the debut of her Podcast in 2018,"Your Marriage Matters," Lynn is committed to helping couples put more sunshine into their marriage. If you value lifelong, happy marriage, you're invited to join the "Your Marriage Matters (YMM) Movement" by signing up on www.marriagecoachlynn.com. You will receive free books as part of the "Your Marriage Matters" series. These titles are exclusive to members of the YMM Movement Group. Visit www.marriagecoachlynn.com to receive your first book in the series, "Make Your Marriage Great: Clean of Heart."

Visit Facebook page (Marriage Coach Lynn), Youtube Channel (Marriage Coach Lynn) and Twitter (MarriageCoachLn). Contact Lynn via email: lynn@bobgriesemer.com or through her websites: www.bobgriesemer.com, www.marriagecoachlynn.com and www.unassistedhomebirth.com.

BOOKS BY LYNN M. GRIESEMER

PUBLIC SPEAKING:

Speak with Ease: Five Secrets Guaranteed to Improve Your Public Speaking Skills (2005, 2017)

"Speak Up! A Public Speaking Program for Young Adults" (2004)

"Speaking Made Easy: A Public Speaking Program for Middle School Students" (2004)

"Public Speaking and Interpersonal Communication" (2006)

MARRIAGE:

Make Your Marriage Great: Clean of Heart (2018)

Reenergize Your Marriage in 21 Days (2011, 2018)

CHILDBIRTH:

Take Back Your Birth: Inspiration for Expectant Moms (2018)

Birthing Unassisted: Another Side of the Story (8/3/18)

Your Body, Your Birth: Secrets for a Satisfying and Successful Birth (CD) (2007)

Unassisted Homebirth: An Act of Love (1998)

The Birth of Your Dreams: How to Have a Successful Birth Experience (2007, 2011)

HUMOR:

Silly Book Titles (2017)

You are invited to post a review of Lynn's books. Your comments are taken seriously and are appreciated.

Made in the USA
Las Vegas, NV
10 September 2023

77399641R00085